YOGA
for Beginners

HARRY WAESSE

YOGA
for Beginners

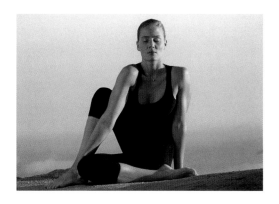

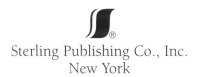

Sterling Publishing Co., Inc.
New York

Contents

Library of Congress Cataloging-in-Publication Data Available

10 9 8 7 6 5 4

Published by Sterling Publishing Company, Inc.
387 Park Avenue South, New York, N.Y. 10016
Originally Published in Germany under the title *Yoga für Anfänger* and © 1995 by Gräfe und Unzer Verlag GmbH, München
English Translation © 1999 by Sterling Publishing Co., Inc.
Distributed in Canada by Sterling Publishing
C/o Canadian Manda Group, One Atlantic Avenue, Suite 105 Toronto, Ontario Canada M6K 3E7
Distributed in Great Britain and Europe by Cassell PLC Wellington House, 125 Strand London WC2R 0BB, England
Distributed in Australia by Capricorn Link (Australia) Pty Ltd. P.O. Box 704, Windsor, NSW 2756, Australia

Printed in Hong Kong
Sterling ISBN 0-8069-2033-5

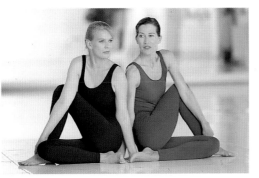

An Important Note

This book is an introduction to yoga. Each reader needs to determine if yoga will be beneficial for him or her. Carry out the exercises only as far as your flexibility will allow—do not force anything. Yoga is based on the principle of "nonviolence," and this important doctrine also plays a role in the way the exercises are performed.

Pay close attention to the instructions, and follow them, step by step. It's also important to observe and not alter the recommended number of repetitions. If you decide that yoga is for you and you want to learn more about it, it would be a good idea to find a yoga class where a qualified teacher can observe your posture and breathing techniques. A class can also be helpful in strengthening the motivation necessary to continue on your "yoga journey."

A Few Thoughts Before You Begin

We live in a hectic world. We rush through each day in order to get everything done. Little time is left to relax and to compensate for daily stress, which is why we so often feel exhausted and overtaxed. Muscles get little attention—we are physically and emotionally tight. Constant physical or emotional tensions rob us of the energies needed to keep well.

Yoga is one of the best ways to deal with tension and to re-energize depleted reserves. Yoga makes us more flexible, physically and mentally, gives us a feeling of being in balance, and helps us live more productive lives. Everyone can get involved in yoga, regardless of age or religious affiliation.

At the beginning, you only do the breathing exercises, because they lead you back to a natural way of breathing, the so-called complete breath. You will find your own breathing rhythm as you get into the physical exercises, the asanas. Yoga breathing, called pranayama, will help you to recharge your energy reserves. Once you are familiar with the breathing exercises, you may begin with the asanas. Because each individual asana has its own distinct effect on the body and the soul, it's important that your yoga program be well balanced. Whether you follow the program in the book or create your own, remember that consistency is the key to success. Exercising every day is best, as this will strengthen your health, improve your flexibility, and give you a sense of peace and tranquility.

The exercises for "in between" allow you to do yoga wherever you are: at work, when traveling, and—when time is short—at home. But no matter where you are, make sure that you won't be disturbed.

The exercises in this book are designed specifically for the beginner. Follow the instructions exactly, and don't overdo it. Take small steps, and you will reach your goal. Experience how yoga gives you an inner peace and serenity, increases your self-confidence, and adds to your physical and emotional well-being.

Harry Waesse

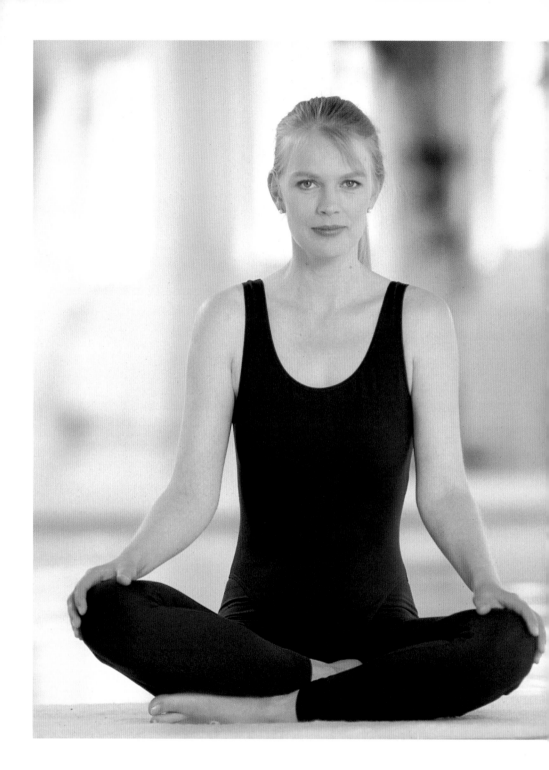

Yoga— the Road to Health

Yoga might well be one of the oldest teachings about life; it was originally taught and promoted by wise men in India, and is practiced today in many different forms, from which anyone may choose according to one's ability and preference.

Should you decide to get involved in hatha yoga, you will find a method of exercising that harmonizes the often opposing energies of body, mind, and spirit. Yoga awakens and promotes the body's own healing powers. Increased health, stamina, balance, and self-confidence are yours for the asking, and are accomplished by combining breathing, physical exercises, and mental concentration. You can only be successful when you learn to combine these three elements.

What Is Yoga?

An ancient method, yoga harmonizes and unites the energies of the human being—the individual self—with the energies of the universe—the higher self. Such harmony, however, can only be achieved if a person is in harmony with him- or herself, or when the energies of body, mind, and spirit are in balance.

Integration of energies

■ According to yoga teachings, the harmony of a person's physical, mental, and spiritual energies means health, whereas their disharmony means illness.

These teachings—stated here in very simple terms intentionally—came from India. Cave paintings and sculptures showing people in obvious yoga positions indicate that yoga has been practiced in India for centuries. Written records about yoga date from the second century B.C., the time when Patanjali, an Indian scientist, began to write down the 195 fundamental rules of yoga. These principles are still accepted to this day. Several different forms of yoga developed from Patanjali's writings, and all are ranked equally.

Yoga—the study of life

■ The yoga exercises presented in this book can bring the energies of body, mind, and spirit into balance, and can be helpful in maintaining or regaining health.

Hatha Yoga—the Way to Harmony

Among the many different forms of yoga practiced today, hatha yoga is the most prominent (*ha* means sun, or the breath of the sun; *tha* means moon, or the breath of the moon). Yoga unites and balances the contrasting energies that we inhale and exhale.

Influencing the whole person

The asanas—a combination of physical movements, breathing, and concentration—influence the whole person in a very positive way: Muscles are strengthened, internal organs and physical movements are harmonized, the circulatory system is stimulated, nerves are calmed, breathing is improved, and concentration is increased.

Life today—with its time, work, and performance pressures and daily conflicts—often leads to physical tension and early wear and tear—even in young people. Psychosomatic illnesses—like stomach problems, diarrhea, and migraine headaches, to name only a few—are not uncommon, and may be the result of physical as well as emotional stress.

■ Hatha yoga can bring definite improvement after practicing it for only a short period of time. It stimulates the healing and strengthening powers of body, mind, and spirit, allowing us to face the demands of everyday life with more equanimity.

Natural, Complete Breathing—Pranayama

Breathing naturally and completely (page 22) provides the body with life-sustaining oxygen (page 18). Although we all did this automatically from day one, most of us seem to have forgotten the "how to" over time. Today, we know that emotional stress and physical tension interfere with the natural process of breathing. Natural, complete breathing is what yoga—with its very specific breathing exercises (page 21)—teaches us. We learn how to breathe properly again. It shows us how to re-establish a natural and harmonious breathing rhythm.

Life-sustaining oxygen

What Is Yoga?

■ Yoga breathing exercises, called pranayama (page 26), require us to master the art of complete, natural breathing. They are meant to recharge depleted energies.

Physical Exercises—Asanas

Central to hatha yoga are the physical exercises, called asanas (page 36). Although the word "asana" means physical exercise, they have nothing to do with exercises in the conventional sense. Asanas are created by combining physical movements with "complete breath" and mental concentration.

A holistic effect Each individual asana uniquely and holistically influences body, mind, and spirit.

Concentration

The third element of hatha yoga is mental concentration, and entails focusing thoughts, emotions, and breath on the area that is being exercised. Concentration engages the body's often conflicting energies.

Opposites attract

■ Once you have mastered the three elements—movement, breath, and concentration—observe how the mind becomes quiet. When yoga is practiced over time, the results include more assertiveness and self-confidence. In addition, previously conflicting internal energies will be in harmony, your reaction to stress (page 13) will be less severe, and your outlook on life will be more positive. As you practice yoga, your "exercise skills" will improve steadily, and the effects will carry over into every aspect of your life.

Yoga and Stress

People often marvel at how such an ancient system as yoga can so profoundly influence the seemingly modern phenomenon of stress. But we tend to forget that stress is as old as life on earth.

What Is Stress?

The word "stress" means pressure. At one point, feeling stressed became synonymous with feeling overwhelmed by the demands of daily life. Today, we know that we need to distinguish between positive stress that is part of normal living and stress that affects us negatively. We all know both!

● Positive stress develops in tension-filled but gratifying situations. Positive stress is often helpful in overcoming old habitual responses and in being more creative, analytical, and imaginative.

Positive stress

Negative stress

● Negative stress is the result of difficult situations. It burdens the system, impedes clear thinking, and alters a person's moods. Being under constant negative stress is known to cause illness.

When we talk about stress in this book, we always refer to the negative kind.

Yoga—the Anti-stress Program

We all know about the negative results of stress: shortness of breath, diarrhea, and headaches, for example. It is now common knowledge that many illnesses are stress-related.

Because each asana—by integrating movement, breath, and concentration—influences body, mind, and spirit, yoga is an ideal way to combat stress and its negative consequences. Physical activity and breathing influence how the body functions, and concentration affects how the mind and the spirit function.

■ Yoga addresses the whole system, and as a result a person is not only better able to deal with stressful situations but also experiences diminished or no negative consequences from them. When yoga exercises are carried out consistently over time, they will bring about a more positive attitude, a relaxed disposition, happiness, and contentment.

Yoga stabilizes

What Is Yoga?

Information about Yoga Worth Knowing

Yoga can be practiced any time and at any age, provided that you are willing to exercise every day. If you are unsure of whether or not yoga is for you, check with your physician.

● You need a large, soft blanket (or yoga mat) for exercising either sitting or lying down. The blanket should be big enough for your size.

● A non-slippery, safe surface is necessary for the exercises you do standing up.

● Do yoga in a large, well-ventilated room. Make sure the temperature in the room is comfortable. It's best to always feel comfortably warm. Exercise outdoors only if the surrounding area is quiet.

● Let nothing distract you: Take the phone off the hook, disconnect the doorbell, and turn off the radio—no music, please.

● Wear comfortable clothing and no shoes when exercising. If you are unable to change into the right clothing, loosen your belt, necktie, and trousers or skirt, and take off your shoes. Also, jewelry, watches, and glasses should be removed.

● Start the yoga routine with the breathing exercises (page 21). Continue with the physical exercises only after you have mastered complete, natural breathing.

● Before starting any of the exercises, read the instructions thoroughly.

● Choose a program (suggestions are listed on page 81), and practice it every day. It is much better to do yoga for 20 minutes every day than to exercise for an hour twice a week.

● Always exercise on an empty stomach, such as in the morning before breakfast. The disadvantage is that you might be still a bit stiff, but the advantage is that you will be refreshed afterward and able to face the events of the day with enthusiasm.

● Should you prefer to do your exercises in the evening or at any other time of the day, eat only a light meal at least two hours before you intend to exercise. This is important, because some of the exercises compress internal organs (stomach and intestines) temporarily.

● This book is written for beginners. It includes many recommendations on how and when to do yoga. It introduces readers to, and familiarizes them with, the series of simple exercises on which yoga is built.

Yoga for beginners

No matter how many photos you look at, or detailed instructions and tips you read, no book is a substitute for an experienced yoga instructor. For this reason, and especially if you want to learn more about and do advanced yoga, enroll in a course. The yoga teacher watches the students' postures and breathing at all times, letting them know if they are doing yoga properly. A class also serves as a motivation to continue on this wonderful journey called yoga.

Take a course in yoga

Observe the Following

Be gentle in the beginning, and find your own rhythm.

Do asana exercises according to your abilities.

Pay attention to warning signs, like nausea, or other discomforts.

Should you experience pain during any of the exercises, stop immediately, go back to the beginning pose, and relax, breathing slowly, quietly, and evenly.

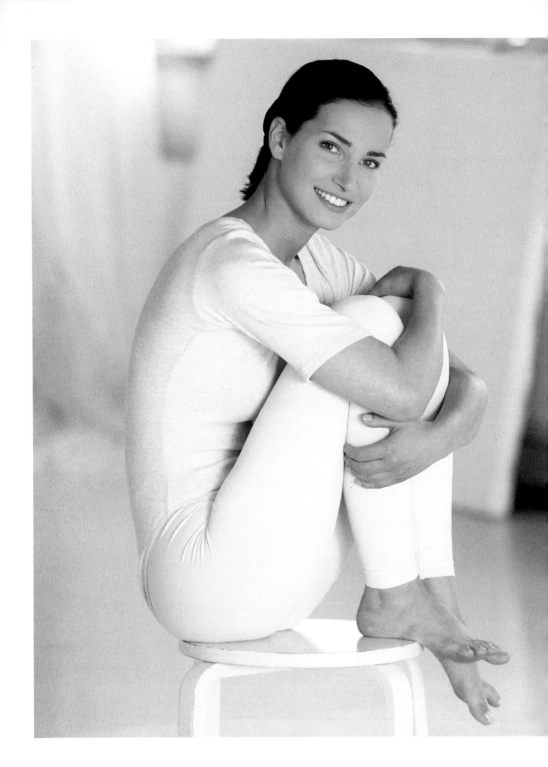

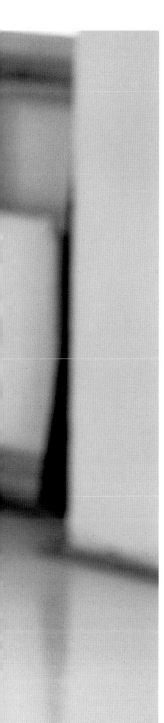

Breath— the Power of Life

Oxygen is important for the different processes that are called metabolism. Only when the breath is deep and relaxed does the body get the oxygen it needs to function properly. This is the reason why complete, natural breathing is such an essential part of doing yoga. Breathing exercises make you conscious of what is essentially an automatic process. The exercises are helpful in finding your own breathing rhythm and in correcting what might possibly be faulty in this regard.

Yoga breathing (pranayama) can recharge your energies and counteract existing health problems. Your body and soul will benefit. You will also become more productive and more balanced.

About Respiration

Breathing is essential for life. Breathing naturally relaxes the body, opens the soul, and clears the mind. Although yoga addresses the whole person in its teachings and practice, it is the process of natural breathing, also called complete or deep breathing, that is of central importance.

Oxygen— Indispensable for Life

Let's first look at the process of respiration, so that you will understand what happens when you breathe in and out, and how much it influences how you feel.

Oxygen is essential for all life-sustaining processes. Without it, you will perish within minutes. When you inhale oxygen-rich air through the nose or the mouth, an exchange of gases inside the tissues of the lungs, called the pulmonary alveoli, is set in motion. Gaseous oxygen enters the bloodstream through the thin walls of tiny blood vessels, transporting it throughout the body to every cell. It is here that oxygen is transformed into energy, which is needed for every phase of metabolism. This process also creates gaseous waste products (carbon dioxide being one of them), which the body needs to get rid of. They are carried by the blood to the pulmonary alveoli and then expelled during exhalation.

■ Respiration is therefore essential for good health and well-being. Only if the process that supplies the body with oxygen by means of inhalation, and expels the waste products by means of exhalation, operates perfectly can you function effectively.

Breathing and the Rhythm of Life

Many of us have forgotten what it means to breathe naturally—the way babies do intuitively. This natural ability has been affected over time by lack of physical exercise, performance pressures, hectic schedules, and the physical and emotional demands of daily life.

Our breath has become shallow, we don't get enough oxygen into the system, and in turn it fails to properly rid the body of its waste products. The result is that we are tired or exhausted and don't feel well or may even be sick.

■ Physical stress and emotional reactions—either negative or positive—also affect the way we breathe. In a sense, breathing is a reflection of a person's physical and mental states, and mirrors the rhythm of his or her life.

When breathing becomes shallow

A Way to Influence Breathing

In order to understand what happens in your body during the breathing exercises, let me briefly explain the physiology of the process. The most important "breathing muscles" are the diaphragm (a bell-shaped muscle plate separating the upper and lower half of the body) and the muscles between the ribs, the intercostal muscles.

● When we inhale, the diaphragm contracts and moves slightly up and down. This motion creates a vacuum in the body and automatically draws air into the lungs. At the same time, the muscles between the ribs lift and expand the ribcage. This increases the capacity of the lungs to take in air, providing the system with more energy-producing oxygen.

● Exhaling is simply a process of relaxation. The diaphragm relaxes, the muscles of the ribcage contract, and air is expelled. This is not a process that is subject to conscious effort—it is automatic.

■ The goal of breathing exercises is to become aware of how we breathe. This will help us find our way back to "complete breathing," something we once knew as babies. It is a way to correct faulty breathing.

Breathing consciously

Breathing Exercises

Yoga breathing exercises make us aware of how we breathe, a process that is essentially automatic. Not only do the exercises help us discover how we are breathing at the moment, but they also influence this process in a positive way. As you gain experience, your breathing will become **Finding** deeper, quieter, and more bal-**your own** anced. You will find your own **breathing** natural rhythm, become more **rhythm** relaxed, and feel better. Breathing naturally will also be helpful during the yoga exercises (asanas). Your breathing rhythm will be more harmonious, and the effect of the exercises more intense. So, start your "yoga journey" with the breathing exercises, paying attention to the following:

■ Take your time as you work with your breath. Don't pressure yourself. Be attentive; get a feeling for and listen to what is going on inside you. Over time, not only will you discover that your breath is influencing the way you do your exercises but also affecting you when you are under pressure and have a special need to stay calm.

Proper Breathing—the Complete Breath

Breathing properly means breathing fully. It is a process in which the diaphragm, the intercostal muscles, and the upper respiratory tract (page 21) work in unison. Only when all three work together do the lungs and the cells receive sufficient oxygen to function at an optimal level, which is necessary for dealing with the waste that is a by-product of the metabolic processes. The stable presence **Oxygen for** of oxygen is beneficial for the **body and** body as well as the spirit: **soul** Consciously breathing with the diaphragm influences physical functions, consciously breathing with the intercostal muscles influences the emotions, and consciously breathing with the upper respiratory tract influences the mind.

● Do the individual breathing exercises ("diaphragm breathing," "breathing with the intercostal muscles," and "top breathing") until you master every aspect effortlessly. Once you have succeeded, practice combining all three.

Breathe through the nose

● Always breathe through the nose. Breathing through the mouth lets dry, unfiltered, and, during the winter months, cold air into the respiratory tract. Too much moisture is withdrawn from your gums, larynx, and the mucous membrane of the respiratory tract. As you inhale, you are more likely to be affected by polluted air and infection-causing germs. Breathing through the nose, on the other hand, cleanses the air as it passes through the nose cavity and its tiny ciliary hairs. Furthermore, the air is warmed by moving past the blood vessels. It also takes up moisture that is present in the sinus cavities.

Diaphragm Breathing

Diaphragm breathing

➤ Start out by lying on your back. Place your right hand on your chest, the left on your navel (photo). Get ready by exhaling. Now inhale deeply, allowing as much air to flow into your lungs as possible. The diaphragm moves down. Feel how the abdominal wall under your hand is lifting. If necessary, press with your right hand against the ribcage so that the chest doesn't expand. Exhale through the nose, as you gently press against the abdominal wall.

● Inhale and exhale 12 times.

● Place your left hand on your chest, and your right hand on your navel, and repeat the same exercise 12 times.

Breathing with the Intercostal Muscles

Breathing with the intercostal muscles

➤ Start by lying on your back. Place your hands at the

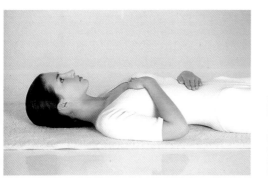

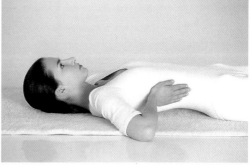

Breathing Exercises

sides of the ribcage, fingers pointing down to the waist **(photo)**. Get ready by exhaling. Now inhale. Imagine that most of the air in your lungs is flowing to both sides of the ribcage. As the chest cavity expands, your hands are pushed out at the sides. Exhale through the nose.

● Start out by doing six of these exercises, and over time increase the number to 10.

Top Breathing

➤ Start by lying on your back. Cross your forearms. Place the right hand on the left upper chest, fingertips touching the collarbone, the left hand on the right upper chest and the fingertips touching the collarbone **(photo)**. Get ready by exhaling. Now inhale. Imagine that most of the air in your lungs

Top breathing

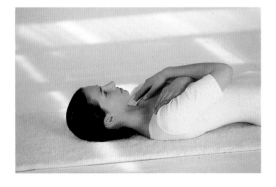

is flowing to the edges and the top of your lungs. The ribcage is expanding, with your hand following the movement. The shoulders should not move up during this exercise. Exhale through the nose. Feel how the upper torso sinks into the floor.

● Start with six top-breathing exercises, and gradually increase to 10.

Complete Breathing

Complete breathing is a combined process involving the diaphragm, the intercostal muscles, and the upper respiratory tract. It is the natural way to breathe, and, over time and with enough experience, will replace faulty breathing.

➤ Start by lying on your back. Concentrate all of your imagination on complete breathing. Begin by exhaling. Then inhale. Feel how the air first fills the lower part of the lungs, lifting the abdominal wall. Notice how the rest of the lungs are filled to capacity, raising the belly and expanding the sides of the flanks and the upper chest. Exhale, allowing the breathing apparatus to relax. Do not exert any extra effort. Over time,

Complete, natural breathing

your breath will become deeper, more even, and longer.

● Start out by doing six complete breaths, and increase the number steadily over time.

Strengthening the Diaphragm

Effects of the exercise: This exercise will strengthen your diaphragm.

➤ Start by lying on your back. Place a book on your belly.

Inhale and exhale deeply

Draw a breath deep into the belly (the book moves up). Exhale (the book moves back to the original position). Increase the weight on your belly every week.

● Do the exercise six to 10 times.

Lengthening Exhalation

Effects of the exercise: This exercise lengthens exhalation without any extra effort.

➤ Start by sitting upright and relaxed on a chair, with the feet and the knees a hips' width apart. The soles of the feet should be in contact with the floor. Hold your upper body upright, and expand the

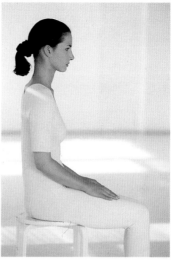

Lengthening exhalation (1)

neck area, feeling how the top of your head is stretching toward the ceiling.

Inhale briefly, while raising the right arm horizontally to shoulder height (photo (**2**), page 24). Exhale, while slowly lowering the right arm back to its original position. Follow the arm movement with your eyes. By concentrating on the movement of the arm, you will automatically and naturally lengthen the duration of exhalation.

● Do the exercise with the right arm three times.

● Do the exercise with the left arm three times.

● Do the exercise with both arms three times.

Breathing Exercises

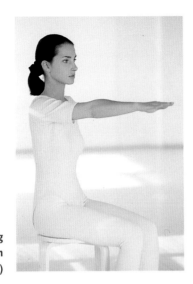

of letters that will make you feel better and that are enjoyable to do.

"Complete breathing" is supported by reciting the vowels u, o, a, e, i while exhaling and by repeating them in your mind while inhaling. In this way, you allow your body to relax from the bottom up, from the pelvis to the head.

Relaxing the body through breathing

● Start with six vocal breathing exercises, and gradually increase to 10.

Vocal Breathing

Effects of the exercise: Including words or sounds during the exercise is another means of lengthening the duration of exhalation. At the same time, the vibrations created by the use of sounds have a relaxing effect on different regions in the body. For instance:
the letter "u" influences the pelvic area,
the letter "o" the waist area,
the letter "a" the chest area,
the letter "e" the throat/neck area, and
the letter "i" the head.

➤ Say or sing the letters individually, while exhaling. Notice the vibrations in your body. Create any combination

Ohm Breathing

Effects of the exercise: Ohm breathing deepens exhalation and relaxes the entire body through the vibrations created by sound.
➤ Start by assuming a relaxed posture. Get ready by inhaling. Now exhale, while making a soft, audible "ohm" sound. Breathe in and out evenly and quietly.

● Do the exercise 10 to 15 times.

■ Pay careful attention to your body, noticing the vibrations of the audible "ohm" in your body. Wherever you can feel the vibration, that is where your body is relaxing.

Ha Breathing

Effects of the exercise: This exercise deepens exhalation, and carbon dioxide and other gaseous waste products are expelled more effectively. It also increases circulation and renews the body's vitality.

Do not do the exercise if there is a danger of retina detachment or internal ocular pressure, or if you have stomach or liver problems or high blood pressure.

▶ Stand upright, with the feet about a shoulders' width apart. Get ready by exhaling. Inhale, while lifting both arms sideways above your head (1).

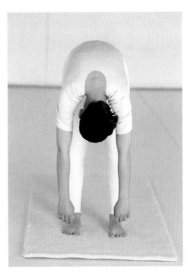

Ha breathing (2)

Exhale, bend at the waist, allowing the upper body to gently fall forward (2), and with a strong voice say "Ha." Return to the upright position, and move the arms vertically over your head.

● Do the exercise three times.

● After the third time, resume the upright position, move the arms vertically over your head, and let them fall down gently as you exhale.

Ha breathing (1)

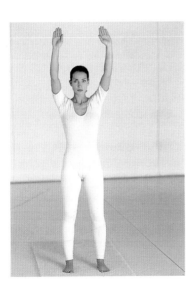

Prana—the Breath of Life

Prana means breath of life, spirit, and vitality. According to yoga teaching, prana is universal energy that is present in all living things.

Prana is vitality, which, together with oxygen, makes breathing such a vital, life-sustaining process. We are all born with a certain potential of prana. The amount of innate prana determines the temperament and the vitality of the individual. If a person has too little prana, he or she will feel tired, listless, weak, and perhaps even sick.

Prana is vitality

The following breathing exercises (pranayamas) can increase prana and thereby improve the quality of your life. You will have more vitality, feel stronger, and experience a greater sense of well-being.

Yoga Breathing— Pranayama

Prana in this context means breathing, and the universal vitality that is our breath; *ayama* means stretching, range, and control. *Prana-yama* is usually translated to mean controlled breathing. Yoga breathing calms the emotions, refreshes the mind, and strengthens the body.

■ Before you start pranayama exercises, you need to have mastered "complete breathing" (page 22).

➤ Pranayama exercises are done sitting. Assume a comfortable position. Always do the pranayama exercises before you start any asanas.

The most important exercise is "alternate breathing." It cleanses the nadis, the energy paths in the body, and should never be omitted. The rest of the pranayama exercises can be integrated into other exercises, depending on how much time you have.

Alternate Breathing

Nadi sodhana: *Nadis* are the paths in the human body (comparable to the meridians that we know from Chinese medicine) through which prana—life's energy—flows; *sodhana* means cleansing and clearing. Alternate breathing cleanses energy paths.

Nadis— energy paths

Effects of the exercise: Alternate breathing cleanses the nadis, the energy paths in the body, balances the flow of prana in the body (for instance, when a person complains about cold feet or cold hands), expands the range of inhalation and exhalation, improves the "breathing process" of each cell (page 18), and relaxes us physically and emotionally.

Do not do these exercises if your nose is congested (you can't breathe through the nose) or if you have not yet mastered "complete breathing."

➤ Sit comfortably in a chair or on a cushion. Keep the upper torso straight, with the shoulders lowered to lengthen the neck, and look straight ahead (photo (1), page 23).

Bend the index and middle finger of the right hand toward the palm of the hand. Press the right thumb against the right side of the nose (1). Exhale and inhale once. Next, with the ring finger of the right hand, close the left side of the nose (2), holding your breath while you switch from the right to the left side, and inhale and exhale once through the right side of the nose.

● Do this breathing exercise, alternating sides, six times, and increase the number gradually over time.

■ The hand position is called vishnu-mudra. *Vishnu* means "preserver of life."

Alternate breathing (1)

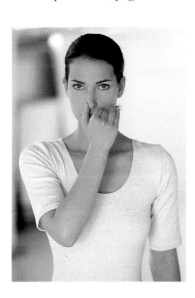

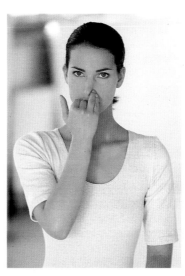

Alternate breathing (2)

Breathing Exercises

Pranayama for Sensitivity to Changes in the Weather

Experience has shown that physical discomfort due to changes in the weather can be prevented with a simplified form of "alternate breathing" (page 26).

Do one of the two exercises described below as early as possible when a drastic change in the weather is forecast. You may do them either lying down or sitting.

Do the exercise as soon as possible

⮞ When you sense a change in the weather—from good to bad—do the "alternate-breathing" exercise as described on page 26 in the following manner: Close the left side of the nose, and inhale with the right side; then switch, closing the right side and exhaling through the left side. Alternate in this way for about two minutes.

● Do the exercise four or five times during the day.

⮞ When you sense a change in the weather—from bad to good—do the "alternate-breathing" exercise as described on page 26. First close the right side of the nose and inhale through the left side.

Then switch, closing the left side and exhaling through the right side. Alternate in this way for about two minutes.

● Do the exercise four or five times during the day.

Cleansing the Brain

Kapalabhati: *Kapala* means skull; *bhati* means light.

Effects of the exercise: This exercise prepares the body to receive prana. It cleanses the body of toxins, stimulates elimination, and reduces fat deposits around the waist. It also stimulates the function of the mucous membrane, cleanses the sinus cavities, and clears the head.

Do not do this exercise if you have heart, lung, stomach, or small-intestines problems, have a tendency toward gallbladder colic, or have recently had surgery.

⮞ Sit comfortably on a chair or a pillow, with the back upright, the shoulders down, and the neck lengthened, and looking straight ahead (photo **(1)**, page 23). Place the palm of the right hand on the stomach, and the left palm on the back of the right hand (**photo**, page 29). Quickly exhale through the

Sit comfortably

nose, while pulling the stomach in and the diaphragm up. Then relax the stomach muscles and inhale passively, which should take about three times as long as the exhalation.

● Do the exercise two times, and increase gradually to six times.

Note: This exercise only involves the diaphragm (page 21); the chest does not move. If you find it difficult to pull the stomach in, you may push with your hands against the abdominal wall.

Bellows Breath

Bhastrika: This means bellows.
Effects of the exercise: Bellows breath refreshes the entire body, removes toxins from the blood and lymph system, stimulates digestion, improves oxygen intake, strengthen nerves, and stimulates the brain.
Do not do the exercise if you have heart, lung, stomach, or small-intestines problems, have a tendency toward gallbladder colic, or have just had an operation.

➤ Sit upright on a chair or a cushion, with the shoulders

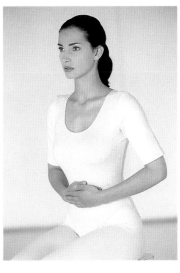

Cleansing the brain through bellows breath

down and the neck long, and looking straight ahead. Place the palm of the right hand on the stomach, and the left hand on the back of the right hand (**photo**). Exhale quickly, while pulling the abdominal wall in and the diaphragm up. Inhale just as fast and through the nose, trying to avoid any kind of effort. The bellow breath is like "complete breathing," except faster.

● Do the exercise two times, and increase the number steadily.

Note: If you have difficulty pulling the stomach in, apply a slight pressure with your hands.

Breathing Exercises for "In Between"

With the following simple breathing exercises, you can improve your oxygen and prana intake and increase your concentration any time during the day. These exercises allow you to regain your natural, harmonious breathing rhythm even in stressful situations. With the help of the "awakening-energies" exercises (page 32), you can create a state of calm, harmony, or strength any time you wish.

Reduce stress

■ These breathing exercises are good to do when you are exhausted or tired, lack concentration, or are nervous— regardless of where you are. You can do them in the office, on a trip, or at home; all that is required is not to be disturbed during the exercise, and to wear clothing that doesn't restrict you in any way. The exercises can also be used as preparation for the standard breathing exercises.

➤ Do the exercises either sitting (photo (**1**), page 23) or standing (photo, page 41).

Both postures allow the breath to flow uninterrupted.

Yawning

Effects of the exercise: The yawning exercise relaxes the muscles in the throat, deepens breathing, supports the elimination of toxins, and dissolves tension.

Unwind

➤ Get ready by exhaling first. Then inhale slowly. Open your mouth, expand the throat, and drop and relax the lower jaw. Then exhale slowly while yawning; at the same time, relax the throat muscles.

● Repeat the yawning several times, while stretching from your fingertips to your toes. Make different sounds during the exercise.

Laughing

Effects of the exercise: It enhances breathing, helps to eliminate toxins, and is a mood-elevator.

Mood-elevator

> Get ready by exhaling first. Inhale slowly. Open your mouth, and during the exhalation say out loud without interruption: "Ha-ha-ha-ha"; at the same time, bend the upper torso forward-this strengthens the effect of the laughing sounds.

Amplify the laughing sounds

● Do the exercise five or six times.

Sniffing Breath

Effects of the exercise: This exercise strengthens exhalation and softens the diaphragm.

> Get ready by exhaling first. Then inhale by sniffing small, even puffs of air. Exhale in one even flow without interruption.

● Start by inhaling with three sniffing breaths, and gradually increase the number, depending on how you feel.

Spreading Fingers

Effects of the exercise: It expands the chest and enhances breathing.

> Get ready by exhaling first. When inhaling, spread and stretch the fingers of both hands. Return the fingers to

their normal position when exhaling.

● Do the exercise five or six times.

Heel Walking

Effects of the exercise: Heel walking stimulates breathing from the diaphragm and relaxes the shoulders, neck, and head.

> Raise your toes, stand on your heels, and take several small steps, while breathing freely.

Heel Raising

Effects of the exercise: Heel raising enhances breathing and strengthens and relaxes the diaphragm.

Relaxes the diaphragm

> Stand upright (page 41). Get ready by exhaling first. As you inhale, raise the heels; as you exhale, lower them again to the floor.

● Do the exercise 15 times.

● Do the same exercise in reverse, also 15 times: Raise your heels as you exhale, and lower them as you inhale.

Praying Hands

Effects of the exercise: It calms and relaxes the entire body.

Place the palms of your hands together in front of your chest, with the fingers pointing upward. Remain in this position for several breaths. Notice how the entire body begins to relax and how your breathing becomes quieter and deeper.

Relaxes the body

This Christian prayer pose and ancient Indian prayer and greeting pose is part of many asanas. The effect can be increased by pushing the hands together while inhaling. Start by applying pressure at the carpal bone, and continue with the palms, then the fingers, and lastly the fingertips. When exhaling, release the pressure in the same sequence, starting at the carpal bone, and so forth.

● Do the exercise three times. Increase the number as you gain experience, depending on how good it feels to you.

Follow Your Breath

Effects of the exercise: This exercise increases concentration, and it teaches you to observe your breathing rhythm without trying to influence it. It is a preparation for "awakening energies" (see below).

Get ready by exhaling first. Inhale, being consciously aware of the air passing from the nose, through the trachea, the air pipe, into the bronchial tubes. Feel the expansion of the lungs. Exhale, feeling how the lungs are emptying out; follow the flow of the air as it leaves the body.

Awakening Energies

The following three exercises are an introduction to the technique of guiding or controlling the energies in the body. It is a technique that will help you awaken your physical, mental, and emotional energies. Depending on the situation, they might address the need for balance, the need for calming the body, or the need to increase your vitality. A prerequisite for the effectiveness of the exercise is concentration (page 40) and the mastery of "complete breathing."

Awakening energies

Smell the Roses

Effects of the exercise: It calms and relaxes body and soul.

▶ Concentrate in your mind on a specific pleasant fragrance. As you inhale, experience this fragrance. Imagine that this wonderful aroma is flowing through your entire body. Exhale, allowing your to breath to move freely and uninhibited.

● Do the exercise from six to 10 times.

Breathing Serenity

Effects of the exercise: This exercise infuses body, mind, and soul with peace and serenity.

▶ Sit upright in a chair (photo (1), page 23). Close your eyes. Exhale and inhale. Observe your breath without trying to influence it. As soon as you are breathing in a quiet rhythm, imagine that with each inhalation you are taking in serenity, peace, and silence. While exhaling, feel how the power of this energy is flow-

ing through your body, mind, and soul. This exercise allows you to summon the energy of harmony, vitality, and other positive states.

● Do the exercise for about 60 seconds.

I Am at Peace

Effects of the exercise: This exercise provides body, mind, and emotions with stillness, balance, and self-confidence.

▶ Sit upright in a chair (photo (1), page 23). Close your eyes. Observe your breathing without trying to influence it. Once your breath is even and flows freely, combine it with the words or thoughts "I am at peace" in the following manner: Concentrate on "I am" while inhaling and on "at peace" while exhaling. This exercise can also be used to awaken any other positive energies, such as harmony or vitality.

Awakens positive energies

● Do the exercise for 60 seconds, and increase the amount of time as you gain experience.

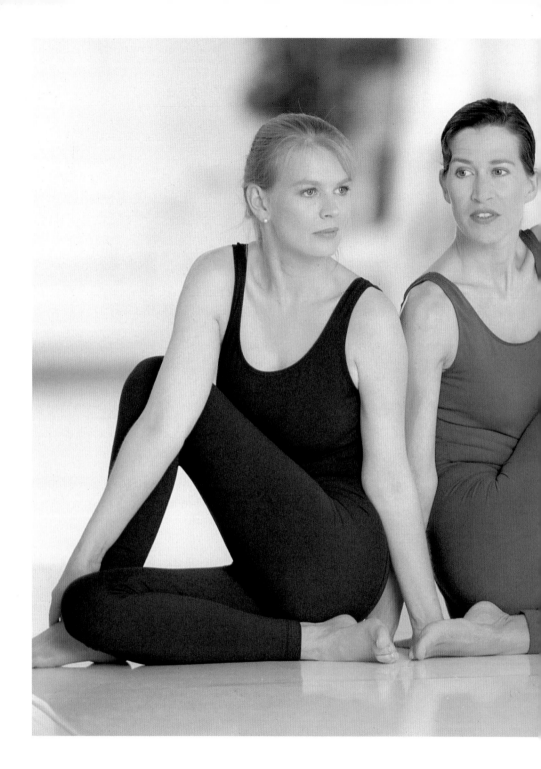

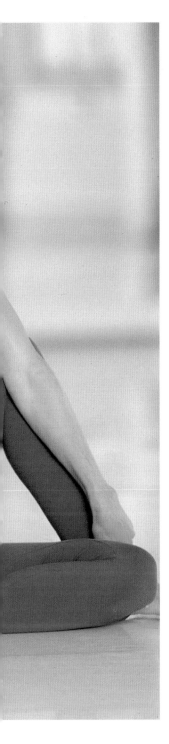

Strengthening Body and Soul

Asana, the yoga exercise, should not be confused with other forms of exercise. It is when breath, concentration, and movement become one that true asana is created. Asanas impact the whole person, with each individual asana having a very specific influence on body, mind, and soul. Therefore, we recommend that you choose a yoga program that you can carry out consistently.

Disregard any and all notions of competition. Exercise only as much as your physical strength allows. Over time and with experience, your physical and mental agility will improve—and your success will be uniquely your own.

About Asanas

The Sanskrit word "asana" originally meant sitting comfortably upright. As hatha yoga began to evolve, the meaning of the word "asana" expanded and became the term for all body positions and physical exercises in hatha yoga.

The effects of asanas

Each asana has a specific influence on body, mind, and spirit. A well-rounded program therefore influences the whole person, including each muscle, nerve, gland, and cell of the body. In addition, practicing hatha yoga asanas is beneficial in other ways. It improves our overall outlook, makes us feel more dynamic and alive, and helps us to find the strength necessary to grow and change. Practicing asanas also gives us more stability, resilience, and patience, as well as a greater sense of peace.

Exercise Phases

Asanas are practiced in four different phases:

● Phase 1: Assuming the starting position

● Phase 2: Guiding the body into the position that is unique to the person

● Phase 3: Remaining in this position

● Phase 4: Returning to the original position

How long a person remains in a particular exercise position (phase 3) depends on the suppleness, the physical strength, and the breath of the individual, as well as on his or her body type.

■ When evaluating your physical strength and flexibility, be realistic. Do each asana the best you can, comfortably. Don't overdo it. Yoga is also called the "path of non-violence," and the principle of non-violence is also very much a part of all the exercises.

Yoga—the path of non-violence

● Move in accordance with your own breathing rhythm,

and pay close attention to how you inhale and exhale.

● Depending on your body type (see below), asanas can be done vigorously or gently, thereby bringing into balance your strengths and weaknesses.

**Compen-
sating for
weaknesses**

Determining Your Type

Before you begin, do some self-analysis. Determine if you belong to the earth type or if you are more of an air type.

■ Characteristics of the earth type: Solidly rooted in the earth, calm, having emotional and physical strength, having persistence, often subject to muscle tension, opinionated, having little imagination, introverted, courageous, dependable.

■ Characteristics of the air type: Less earth-bound, active, adaptable, creative, imaginative, having little muscular strength, physically and emotionally volatile, tending toward superficiality, having limited stamina, extroverted, fearful.

■ The earth type should do the asanas vigorously, because

the exercises will help to dissolve tensions.

➤ Proceed as follows: Assume your personal exercise posture as you inhale. Remain in that position for a few breaths, and then return to the starting position as you exhale. This will dissolve tensions and increase physical and emotional suppleness. You will begin to "open up" and be more flexible.

■ It's best for the air type to perform the asanas more gently, because the exercises are an opportunity to practice patience, develop stamina, become calmer, and increase vitality.

**Developing
patience
and stamina**

➤ Assume your personal exercise posture as you inhale. Remain in this position for a few breaths, to stretch the more deeply seated muscles. This will increase vitality, improve posture, and dissolves tensions. Return to the starting position during the exhalation.

■ Should you feel that you are a combination of the earth and air types, alternate between the two forms of exercise. A few asanas always have to be done in the more gentle

About the Asanas

form, regardless of your body type. Pay close attention to the instructions for the individual exercises.

Characteristics of Asanas

According to Patanjali (see page 10), each asana should be correct and carried out with lightness and comfort.

The Accuracy of Asanas

Each asana should have a firm foundation and be accurate. The posture from which each movement emanates, and the way you move from the starting position to your (personal) exercise posture and back again, must be carried out with as much care as possible.

● The earth type should balance and energize accuracy with enthusiasm. (See page 37.)

● The air type needs to soften intensity with calmness. (See page 37.)

The Lightness of Asanas

Lightness is a happy state, falling somewhere between

severity and dissolution. You will be able to find the lightness of the exercises when you first do them in your imagination.

➤ Assume the starting position, and, with your eyes closed, exercise in your mind without moving a muscle. Pay close attention to the way your breathing rhythm and muscle tone changes. This awareness is the basis for self-control and successful improvements. But this visualizing exercise also points out how much our bodies tend to exaggerate. Our bodies always want to invest more energy than necessary, and this interferes with breathing.

● Repeat the visualization exercise, and try to integrate the rhythm of your breath with the muscle tone.

● Next, do the exercise physically, incorporating the experience of the visualization.

The Comfort of Asanas

In the beginning, many of the exercises will be anything but comfortable. You may only be able to do many of asana movements partially, or may have trouble doing them at all, because you aren't yet flexible enough. But with regular exercising, you will loosen stiff muscles and find your flexibility restored or improved over time. Ever-increasing flexibility will be one of your rewards. You may be relieved to know that improvement in physical agility is preceded by improvement of the mental and emotional states, because yoga balances the human system from the subtle to the more coarse areas of the body.

Yoga harmonizes the human system

Please Take Note

Yoga restores natural flexibility. If the body is overtaxed by impatient or careless movements, this can result in pulled muscles and/or overstretched tendons—a sure sign that the person wants to do more than his or her body is capable of handling. Once you have discovered "the middle of the road," the place between rigidity and dissolution, you will do the exercises accurately and with ease and comfort.

Active Stretching

Active stretching is the best way to achieve accuracy, ease, and comfort. Active stretching involves visualizing extending the reach of the activated muscles in specific areas. Here is an example:

➤ Assume the "upright position" (see page 41). Imagine that you are exploring your body from the top of your head down to the end of the spine, from the shoulders down the arms to the tips of the fingers, and from the heels to the toes. Shift your weight to the right foot. Place the instep of the left foot over the right foot. Hold the hands with the palms together in front of you, the fingers pointing upward.

Now imagine the tips of your fingers becoming longer and longer. Inhale and lift the arms and the "elongated" fingers above your head (**photo**, page 43, right). Then in your mind's eye explore once more, starting at the tips of the fingers, going down to the end of the spine, and going past the heels to your toes. This is what is meant by active stretching.

Use your imagination

About the Asanas

The body will only activate the muscles necessary for the exercise, the breath will flow unhindered, and physical and emotional tensions will dissolve.

Dissolving tension

Asanas and Concentration

Concentration here refers to the ability of body, spirit, and mind to be engaged in the exercises in equal measure. Over time, this will lead to an increasingly harmonious, conscious interaction of the whole person. Concentration deepens physical awareness and awakens a feeling for the flow of movements during the exercises. The result is a life lived in a more balanced way.

Asanas and Breathing

During the exercises, breathe consciously, deeply, and steadily, and in a relaxed manner.

● Breathing consciously means developing an awareness of the life-sustaining process that we usually take for granted. It means observing the motion, depth, and rhythm of breathing, and working toward achieving "complete breathing" (see page 22). This in turn will improve vitality, strength, awareness, and concentration.

● Natural, complete breathing means that all organs and areas of the body are involved in the breathing process; the diaphragm and the muscles on both the sides and the upper part of the body (see pages 21 and 22) are actively and effortlessly engaged.

● Relaxed breathing means allowing all the muscles involved in the process to relax naturally during inhalation. Breathe "silently." Make sure that the muscles in the shoulder, chest, and pelvic areas are not engaged but kept relaxed. To do otherwise would interfere with the natural breathing process. Consciously experience exhalation as relaxation.

Conscious relaxation

● Rhythmic breathing means to observe the length, depth, and ease when exhaling and inhaling. Quiet inhalation should be followed by a slightly longer exhalation. If possible, and if you are feeling well, pause briefly after each exhalation.

Asanas—Exercises

What follow are a series of simple exercises called asanas. In order to avoid repetition, the exercises are organized according to their respective starting position and degree of difficulty rather than by exercise programs.

● We have listed eight exercise programs on pages 81 through 83, so that you don't to have to put together your own program. The first program is the easiest, with each subsequent program becoming progressively more difficult. Start with Program I. Practice it regularly, preferably every day. Once you feel comfortable and are familiar with the program, proceed to the next one.

Follow all instructions

● If you want to put together your own program, start with the easy and simple exercises.

■ Take note of the alternative positions mentioned in the instructions.

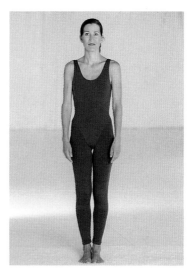
Upright position

Upright Position

Tadasana: *Tad* means mountain. Tadasana is a posture in which you stand upright with your feet planted solidly on the ground.

This is the basic posture for all asanas that evolve from standing upright.

Effects of the exercise: The upright position provides relief for the spine, joints, muscles, and tendons. Shoulder and back problems, due to poor posture, can be

Asanas—Exercises

Gaining strength and courage

either lessened or prevented. Standing with both feet solidly on the ground fosters courage, strength, and self-confidence.

▶ Stand upright, with the feet close together and the weight balanced equally on both heels, balls, and toes of the feet.

The kneecaps are pulled up slightly by tensing the thigh muscles.

The back is straight, not hollow (see **photo**, page 41).

Feel the chest move out barely, while letting the shoulders and the arms sink down and slightly back.

Gently extend the neck, and let the top of your head become aware of the space above it.

Breathe quietly and evenly throughout the exercise.

Pendulum

Effects of the exercise: The pendulum improves circulation in the head and the upper body, relieves tension in the shoulders, and improves posture.

▶ Assume the "upright position" (page 41), but with the feet about 11 in., or 30 cm, apart and the left hand resting at the waist.

During exhalation, bend the upper torso forward at the hips into a horizontal position. Allow the right arm to swing in front of the legs without exerting any effort physically or mentally **(1)**. Breathe quietly and evenly throughout the exercise. Move the right arm up and as far back as possible (photo **(2)**, page 43). Give the arm a good stretch, and then allow it to "fall" down again.

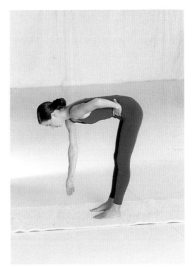

Pendulum (1)

**Pendulum
(2)**

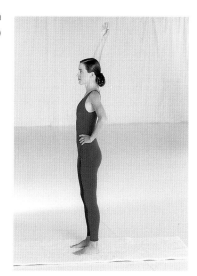

muscles; push the pelvis to the left.

Place the sole of the right foot over the left instep, with the heel facing the outside; the toes do not touch the floor. Put the palms of the hands together in front of the upper body, the fingers pointing upward. As you inhale, move your arms above your head **(photo)**. Hold this posture for a few breaths.

Stretch the upper body upward from the pelvis. Inhale and lower the arms.

● Repeat the exercise with the left arm, and then with both arms.

● Repeat the entire sequence two or three times.

● Do this exercise, alternating sides, for two to three minutes.

Tree Pose I

Vrksasana: *Vrksa* means tree.

Effects of the exercise: It supports breathing and improves stability, balance, and concentration.

➤ Assume the "upright position," with the feet together (page 41). Shift the weight to the left leg, stabilizing the left knee and the hip joints by contracting the thigh

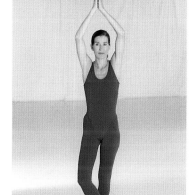

Tree (1)

Asanas—Exercises

Squat I (1)

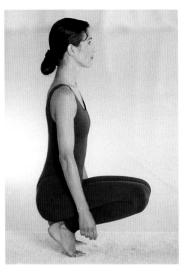

Squat I (2)

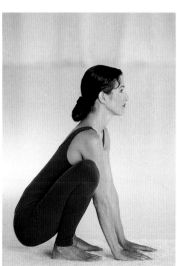

Squat I

Utkasana: *Utkata* means powerful.

Effects of the exercise: This exercise strengthens the feet and toes, is beneficial for sunken arches, and prevents varicose veins. It also supports the sense of balance.

➤ Assume the "upright position" (page 41), but with the feet about 7 to 11 in. (20 to 30 cm) apart.

Squat down until you are sitting on the heels, and lift the heels off the floor, shifting the weight to the toes (**1**).

Slowly lower the feet until the soles are flat on the floor. Allow the seat to sink as far down as possible, and lay the hands flat on the floor (**2**). Now shift the weight back to the toes, and slowly assume the "upright position." Breathe in a relaxed manner and evenly throughout the exercise.

● In the beginning, repeat the exercise three times. Increase the repetitions up to eight times, as you gain experience and strength.

Leaning Half-Moon

Parsva-ardha-chandrasana:
Parsva means leaning to the
side, *ardha* means half, and
chandra means moon.

Effects of the exercise: It
stretches the neck, shoulder,
arm, pelvis, and leg muscles,
stimulates digestion, increases
flexibility, reduces fat deposits
under the skin, and creates
more harmony between the
upper and lower body.

Do the exercise with extra
care if you have back or
spine problems or problems
Important! with the muscles between the
ribs.

Do not do this exercise
right after surgery or if you
have intestinal inflammation.

➤ Assume the "upright
position," with the feet
together (page 41).

Raise both arms over your
head while inhaling; put your
palms together, or hook your
thumbs together, with the
palms held away from the
body **(1)**.

Now stretch upward, imag-
ining that the fingertips are
moving further and further
up.

Exhale as the pelvis is
pushed to the right and the
upper body to the left, all the
time holding the stretch. The
head is facing straight ahead
(2). Remain in this position
for three or four breaths.

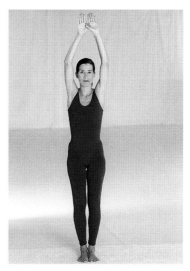

Leaning
half-moon
(1)

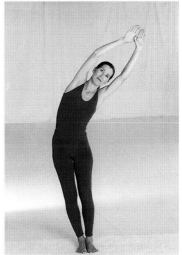

Leaning
half-moon
(2)

**Hold the
stretch**

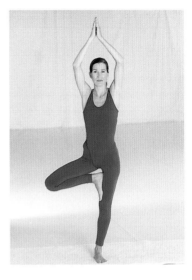

Asanas—Exercises

Inhale and move back to the center, with the arms still held overhead. Begin to stretch upward again. Exhale and shift the pelvis to the left and the upper body to the right; hold the stretch.

● Repeat, alternating sides; do two or three repetitions on each side.

Tree II

Tree Pose II

Vrksana: *Vrksa* means tree.
    Effects of the exercise:
It improves balance and strengthens the muscles of the feet, legs, and shoulder area.

➤ Assume the "upright position," with the feet to-gether (page 41).
    Shift the weight to the left foot. Place the sole of the right foot against the inside of the left leg above the knee. Put the palms together in front of the upper body, and move the arms slowly above the head.
    Turn the bent knee to the outside as far as possible, preferably in line with the right shoulder **(photo).**

Imagine reaching further and further to the sky with the fingertips, and further and further down from the pelvis all the way to the heels. Remain in this position for 20 to 30 seconds.
    Slowly lower the arms to chest height; then let them sink down to the sides, as you return the right foot to the floor.
    Repeat the exercise with the left foot.

● Do the exercise, alternating sides, twice on each side.

Side Triangle

Utthita-trikonasana: *Utthita* means spreading out, *trikona* triangle.

Effects of the exercise: The side triangle strengthens the pelvic and leg muscles, stretches the spine, and stimulates the functions of the liver, gallbladder, and pancreas.

Do not do the exercise if you have hip problems or problems in the intercostal region.

Important!

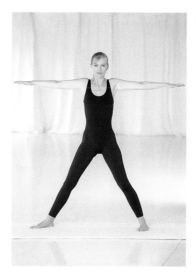

Side triangle
(1)

➤ Assume the "upright position" (page 41). Depending on your size, place your feet 27 to 39 in. (70 to 100 cm) apart.

Raise the arms straight out to shoulder height, while inhaling—palms down. Turn the right foot about 90 degrees and the left foot 15 degrees to the right (**1**). Exhale as you bend the upper body to the right, with the right arm extending down and the left arm up. Look at your left thumb (**2**). Retain the position for 30 seconds. Inhale as you assume the "upright position" (**1**).

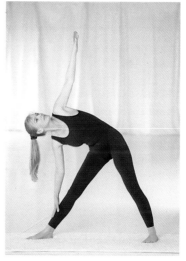

Side triangle
(2)

● Do this exercise, alternating sides, for two to three minutes.

Twisting Triangle

Parivrtta-trikonasana:
Parivrtta means reverse,
trikona triangle.

Effects of the exercise: The
effects are like those of the
"side triangle" (page 47).
Twisting in the waist mobilizes the back and spine.

➤ Assume the "upright
position" (page 41). Inhale
and move the feet about 27 to
39 in. (70 to 100 cm) apart.

Raise the arms straight out
to the sides, palms down.

Exhale, while bending the
upper body at the hips; the
back and arms remain horizontal (**1**).

Turn the upper body so
that the palm of the right
hand can be placed at the
outside of the left calf or
ankle. Look up at the left
hand (**2**). Remain in this position for about 10 seconds,
breathing calmly and evenly.

Inhale and lift the upper
body and arms back to the
horizontal position (**1**). Exhale; with the next inhalation,
move back to the "upright
position."

Practice with the other
side.

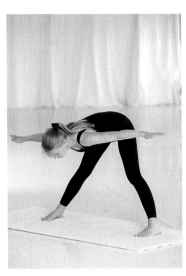

**Twisting
triangle (1)**

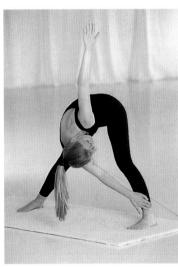

**Twisting
triangle (2)**

● Do the exercise four times on each side, alternating sides.

Squat II

Utkasana: *Utkata* means powerful.

Effects of the exercise: They are the same as for "squat I" (page 44).

Important!

Do not do the exercise if you have pain in the knee joints.

➤ Assume the "upright position" (page 41).

Inhale, raising the arms horizontally in front of the body.

Exhale, squatting down, feet together, until the soles of the feet are flat on the floor.

Inhale and lift the heels, shifting the weight to the toes. Next, sit back on the heels and place both hands on the knees **(photo)**. Remain in this position for about 20 seconds, breathing calmly and evenly.

Go back to the "upright position" by reversing the order of the sequence.

● Repeat the exercise three times. Increase the repetitions up to eight times, as you gain experience and strength.

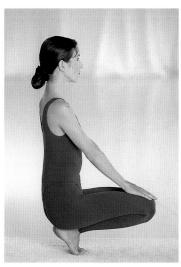

Squat II

Hero

Virabhadrasana: *Virabhadra* means big hero.

Effects of the exercise: They are the same as for the "side triangle" (page 47). In addition, bending mobilizes the back and spine, strengthens the leg, shoulder, and arm muscles, increases circulation in the lower half of the body, and supports the function of the colon.

➤ Stand upright (page 41).

Hero (1), (2)

Inhale, placing the feet 27 to 39 in. (70 to 100 cm) apart, while lifting the arms straight out to the sides to shoulder height, palms facing down (1). Turn the right foot approximately 90 degrees and the left foot 15 degrees to the right. Exhale as you move the right knee to the right, until the calf is in a vertical position. The left leg remains where it was. The right foot and right hand point in the same direction. Look at the right hand (2). Remain in this position for about 15 to 20 seconds, breathing calmly and evenly.

Reverse the order of the movements, until you reach the starting position again.

● Do the exercise twice on each side.

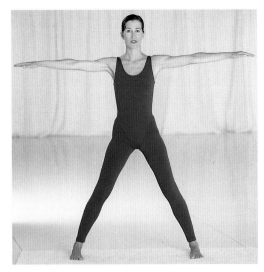

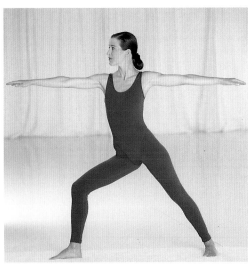

Stretched Hand-Toe Pose

Utthita-hasta-padangustha-asana: *Utthita* means stretched out, *hasta* means hand, and *padangustha* means big toe.

Effects of the exercise: It strengthens the arm and leg muscles, and increases the sense of balance.

Do not do the exercise if your sense of balance is impaired.

Important!

➤ Assume the "upright position" (page 41).

Shift the body weight to the left knee. Inhale, while pulling the right foot up along the inside of the left leg, holding the foot at the big toes with the thumb and the index and middle finger of the right hand. Place the left hand at the hip (**1**). Remain in this position for three breaths, or until you feel well balanced. Now exhale as the right leg is stretched forward (**2**). Remain in this position for the length of two to three breaths.

Exhale and reverse the order of the movements, until you reach the starting position again.

● Do the exercise, alternating between sides, twice on each side.

**Stretched
hand-toe
pose (1)**

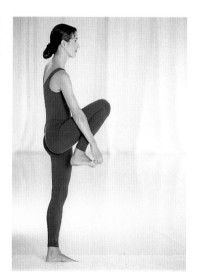

**Stretched
hand-toe
pose (2)**

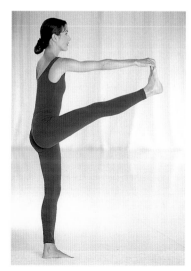

Full Bend

Uttasana: *Ut* means upward, as well as intense and gentle; *tan* means stretching and elongating.

Effects of the exercise: The full bend stretches the back muscles, stimulates the functions of the pancreas, liver, and kidneys, increases blood circulation in the head, improves mental activity, and lengthens exhalation.

Asanas—Exercises

Do not do the exercise if there is a danger of high ocular pressure or retina detachment, or if you have back problems or high blood pressure.

Conclude with the "corpse-pose stretch" (page 70) or "shoulder bridge" (page 71).

➤ Assume the "upright position" (page 41), with the feet a hips' distance apart.

Exhale, while the stretched upper body bends forward as far as possible at the hips (the upper body should be at a right angle to the legs); the arms are relaxed and hanging down (1). Breathe evenly and calmly. With each exhalation, bend the upper body, vertebrae by vertebrae, further down, until you can reach the floor in front of the toes with the fingertips or the palms of the hands. With each inhalation, move the head and upper body ever so gently closer and closer to the legs. Depending on your flexibility, grasp the calves or ankles (2). Remain in this position for one to two minutes. Breathe deeply and evenly. Inhale and gradually lift the upper body in reverse order back into the horizontal position.

With the next inhalation, return to the starting position.

● Do the exercise two or three times.

**Full bend
(1)**

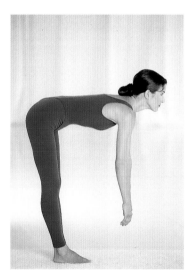

**Full bend
(2)**

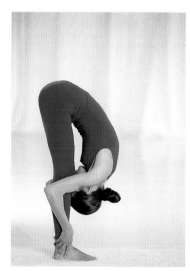

● Suggestion: If the fingers or hands cannot reach the floor in the beginning, place the hands on another surface, such as a low stool.

Knee Stand

This is the position for all exercises that evolve from the kneeling position.

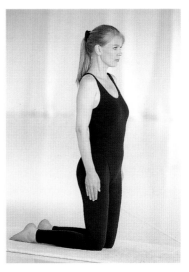

Knee stand

➤ Stand upright (page 41).
Next, kneel down on a soft surface, with the instep of the feet flat on the floor. Have your body weight divided equally between both knees.
Place the right hand at the end of the spine, and the left hand on the belly below the navel. With the right hand, push the pelvis forward, with the left hand back. The thighs remain straight and upright.

Straighten the back and chest, allowing the shoulders to sink down and back; the arms remain relaxed at the sides.
Stretch the neck, and pull the chin slightly in the direction of the chest **(photo).**

Asanas—Exercises

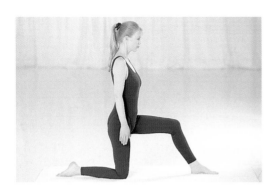

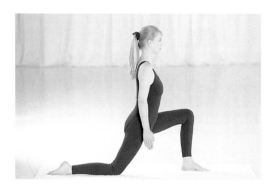

Half-cobra
(1), (2) *Half-Cobra*

Ardha-bhujangasana: *Ardha* means half, and *bhujanga* means serpent or cobra.

Effects of the exercise: The half-cobra strengthens the back muscles, stretches the muscles at the front of the body and the thighs, strengthens the lower back and the hip joints, reduces fat deposits in the hips and thighs, loosens the shoulder region, stimulates kidney function, and helps to lower blood pressure.

Do not do the exercise if you have lower-back or hip problems, if there is inflammation in the abdomen or the uterus, after a recent operation, or when recovering from a fracture. **Important!**

Conclude with the "corpse-pose stretch" (page 70).

➤ Assume the "knee stand" (page 53).

Place the left foot in front of you; the angle between the thigh and the calf should be slightly more than 90 degrees. The shoulders and arms are relaxed and down **(1)**.

Concentrate on the back of the pelvis as you exhale, pushing the pelvis forward as far as possible; the upper body remains upright **(2)**. Stay in this position for four breaths, stretching the body from the top of the head all the way to the tips of the toes of the right foot.

Return to the "knee stand," and repeat the exercise with the other leg.

● Do the exercise, alternating legs, two or three times on each side.

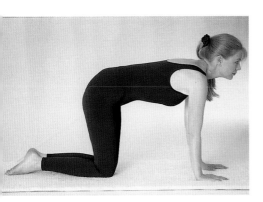

Dog pose

Dog Pose

Effects of the exercise: It relieves and strengthens the shoulder and hip joints.

➤ Assume the "knee stand" (page 53). Bend the upper body forward, and rest the weight of the arms on the palms of the hands on a floor mat, the fingers pointing forward **(photo)**.

Cat

Effects of the exercise: The cat increases the flexibility of the back and shoulder muscles and the hips, tightens tissue and reduces fat

deposits in the waist, stomach, and seat, stimulates the digestive organs, and counteracts fatigue.

Do not do the exercise if you have spinal injuries or severe pain in the shoulders, hips, or knees.

Conclude with the "corpse-pose stretch" (page 70).

➤ Assume the dog pose (left); the hands are a shoulders' width apart, the knees a hips' width apart.

Exhale, rounding the back, letting the head sink forward, and pulling the right leg to the chin **(1)**.

Inhale, returning the back to a straight position, stretching the right leg out and up, and moving the head back; stretch the entire body (photo **(2)**, page 56).

Cat (1)

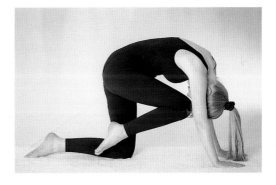

Asanas—Exercises

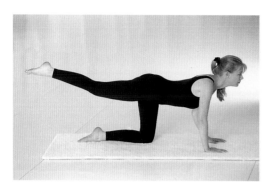

Cat (2)

Heel-Seat Position

This is the basic position for all exercises evolving from it.

Effects of the exercise: It strengthens the feet and legs, and improves circulation in the pelvic and abdominal areas.

Do not do the exercise if you have varicose veins or knee or ankle injuries.

➤ Assume the "knee stand" (page 53); the heels are turned to the outside.

Bend forward, assuming the "dog pose" (page 55). Place the fingertips on the sides of the knees, and balance your weight evenly between the arms and the legs. Lower your buttocks, and sit in the space between your legs.

As soon as the buttocks are securely placed on your feet, place the palms of the hands on the thighs. Sit with the pelvis and the back upright and the shoulders comfortably down and back **(photo)**. Imagine the top of your head reaching (gently) upward.

● Do the exercise twice.

● Suggestion: As an aid, you might want to place a pillow under the ankle joints or the buttocks.

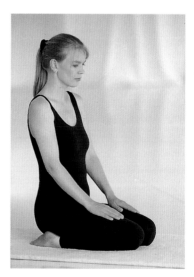

Heel-seat position

Baby Pose

Effects of the exercise: The baby pose stretches and relaxes tension in the shoulder and back muscles, improves circulation in the brain, calms the nervous system, deepens breathing, and reduces stress.

Do not do the exercise if you have varicose veins, pain in the hips, knees, or ankles, or injuries to the spine.

Conclude with the "corpse-pose stretch" (page 70).

➤ Assume the "heel-seat position" (page 56).

Bend the upper torso forward until your head touches the floor. At the same time, move the arms back, placing the backs of the hands alongside the calves. The upper body and the head are completely relaxed **(photo).**

The baby pose is a relaxing, humbling position that can be maintained for a longer period of time than the other positions. The breathing is calm and even throughout the exercise.

Return to the "heel-seat position" by first moving the upper body and then the

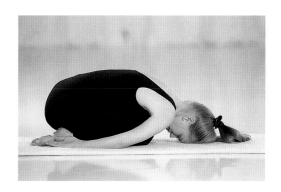

Baby pose

head. Bring the head upright only after the upper body is in an upright position.

● Do the exercise once.

Lion

Simhasana: *Simha* means lion.

Effects of the exercise: The lion relaxes the face and smoothes out wrinkles. It also strengthens the voice and is helpful if you have a sore throat.

➤ Assume the "heel-seat position" (page 56). The toes are on the mat, the back is straight, the palms are on the thighs, the arms are stretched slightly, and the fingers are spread out (photo **(1)**, page 58).

Lift the buttocks off the heels. Lean the upper body forward, letting the hands slide down and the fingers rest under the knees. Then open the mouth, push the tongue down to the chin, and look at the tip of the nose (**2**). Remain in this position for 10 seconds, inhaling and exhaling through the mouth.

● Do the exercise twice.

Flower

Effects of the exercise: The flower relaxes stiff fingers, eases joint pain, improves circulation in the hands, and warms cold hands.

➤ Assume the "heel-seat position" (page 56). Lift the forearms so that the hands are shoulders' height, and make tight fists (photo (**1**), page 59).

Imagine that your hands are flowers that slowly unfold, and continuously "push against" the unfolding. Stretch the fingers as far as possible (photo (**2**), page 59). With the same force, make tight fists again.

Then open the fists once more and jiggle the hands and fingers.

● Do the exercise three times.

Lion (1)

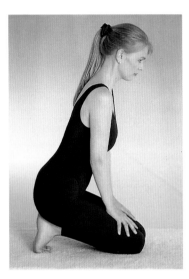

Lion (2)

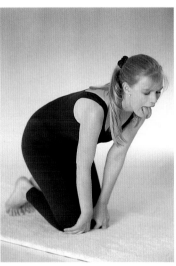

Flower (1)

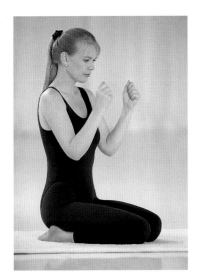

Blade (1)

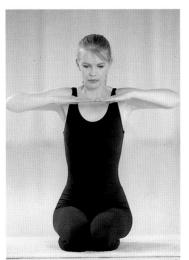

Flower (2)

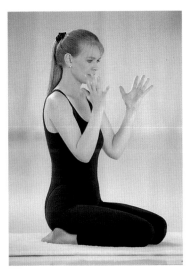

Blade

Effects of the exercise: It strengthens the shoulder muscles and joints, eases shoulder tension, firms the chest muscles, and deepens breathing.

➤ Assume the "heel-seat position" (page 56). Stretch out the arms, and lift them to shoulders' height. Bend the forearms so that the hands are in front of the chest, with the palms pointing down and the fingertips touching (1).

Blade (2)

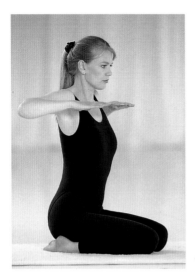

Push the shoulder blades together, with the arms following the movement passively (2). Remain in this position for 10 seconds, dissolving the tension in the shoulder region and the back.

● Do the exercise five times.

➤ Next, push the elbows back, keeping the arms and hands horizontal. From the shoulder joints, move the arms up and down five to eight times.

● Do this three times.

Seated Sun Pose

This is the basic position for exercises evolving from the sitting position on the floor.

Effects of the exercise: The seated sun pose relaxes muscle tension in the pelvis, back, shoulders, and neck.

➤ Sit on a mat or a pillow with the legs extended. Place the palm of the right hand under the right sitting bone. Pull the hand back and out (this moves the pelvis upright). Do likewise on the left side. Make sure that the weight of the body is distributed equally between both sides of the pelvis.

Seated sun pose

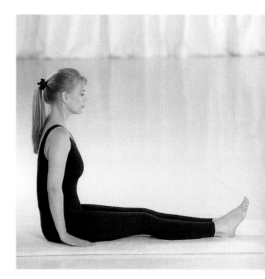

Straighten the back and the chest; the shoulders are down and slightly pulled back.

Drop the shoulders, and pull them back slightly. Stretch the neck, and move the chin down in the direction of the chest (**photo**, page 60).

Increasing Flexibility

Effects of the exercise: It stretches the muscles of the back, groin area, and legs.

Do not do the exercise if you have pain or pulled ligaments in the groin region or a hernia.

Increasing flexibility

➤ Assume the "seated sun pose" (page 60).

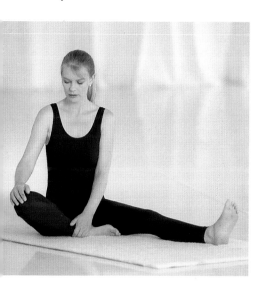

Place the sole of the right foot as high as possible against the inside of the left thigh. Gently hold the ankle of the right foot.

Place the right hand on the right knee, and gently push the knee to the floor in a bouncing motion (**photo**). The breath is relaxed and even.

If the knee makes contact with the floor—with the upper torso remaining straight—you have achieved the goal of the exercise.

● Do each side six to eight times, starting with the right leg.

Tailor's Seat

Sukhasana: *Sukha* means effortless.

Effects of the exercise: It stretches the muscles of the pelvis, groin area, and legs, strengthens the back, and prepares one for other sitting positions.

Do not do the exercise if you have pain or pulled ligaments in the groin region or a hernia.

Important!

Asanas—Exercises

Tailor's seat

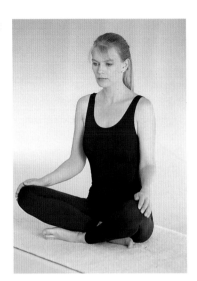

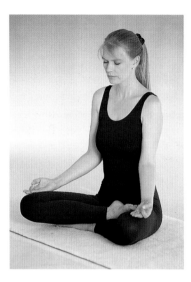

➤ Assume the "seated sun pose" (page 60).

Place the sole of the right foot as high as possible against the inside of the left thigh. Place the left heel under the right calf.

Place the hands on the knees (**photo,** above left). You may also place the backs of the hands on the knees with the thumbs and index fingers touching (**photo,** above right).

● This is a meditation pose called jnana-mudra that deepens concentration.

Meditation Pose

Muktasana: *Mukti* means freedom.

Effects of the exercise: It stretches the muscles of the pelvis, groin area, and legs, straightens the back, and relaxes the neck and shoulders; the jnana-mudra position of the hands is a meditation pose.

Do not do the exercise if you have pain or pulled ligaments in the groin area or a hernia.

➤ Assume the "seated sun pose" (page 60). Pull the left heel to the perineum, and the right heel in front of the left ankle. Both knees sink gently to the floor.

Place the right hand under the right sitting bone; pull the hand back toward the outside. Do likewise on the left side. This will move the pelvis to an upright position, and the knees will sink even deeper into the floor. Place the back of the hands on the knees; the tips of the thumbs and the index fingers are touching, and the rest of the fingers are straight (jnana-mudra, **photo** on page 62, right). The breath is relaxed and even.

Meditation pose

You may also place the back of the left hand on the foot, and the back of the right hand on top of the palm of the left hand with the tips of the thumbs touching (dhyana-mudra).

● Do the exercise, alternating sides, two or three times on each side.

● Suggestion: Sit on a firm pillow.

Mountain Variation

Parvatasana: *Parvata* means mountain.

Effects of the exercise: It strengthens the shoulder and arm muscles, deepens breathing, improves oxygen intake, and strengthens the spine.

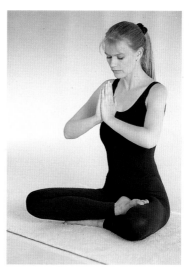

Mountain variation (1)

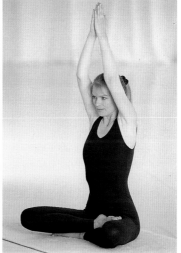

Mountain variation (2)

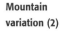 Assume the "meditation pose" (page 62). Sit upright and place the palms of the hands together, holding them in front of the chest (**1**).

Asanas—Exercises

Inhale, moving the arms above the head (photo **(2)**, page 63). The tips of the fingers stretch upward, and the sitting bones stretch down into the floor. Allow the breath to flow freely. Remain in this position for about 10 to 15 seconds. Exhale, returning the arms to the original position in front of the chest.

● Do the exercise twice.

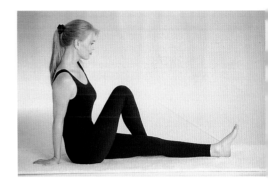

Half Spinal Twist

Ardha-matsyendrasana: *Ardha* means half; *Matsyendra* is the founder of hatha yoga.

Effects of the exercise: The half spinal twist stretches the back muscles, relieves tension in the neck and shoulders, stimulates the functions of the liver, stomach, and pancreas, increases the flexibility of the hip joints, strengthens the nervous system, and harmonizes organ flow.

Important! Exercise with care if you have pain in your back or hips.

Conclude with the "corpse-pose stretch" (page 70) or "shoulder bridge" (page 71).

➤ Assume the "seated sun pose" (page 60).

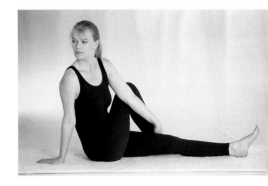

Half spinal twist (1), (2)

Bend the right leg, keeping the right foot resting on the mat; then place right foot parallel to the outside of the left knee **(1)**. Turn the head, upper torso, and arms to the right, placing the right hand on the floor behind the buttocks for support.

Hold the outside of the right ankle with the left hand; the left upper arm pushes the right knee to the outside.

Look back over the right shoulder; the breath is relaxed and even, and both sitting bones remain in contact with the floor (photo **(2)**, page 64).

● Do the exercise, alternating sides, two or three times on each side.

Leg Stretch

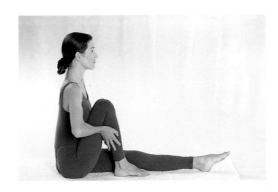

Effects of the exercise: It stretches the muscles of the lower back, buttocks, and legs, compensates for a hollow back, and improves the mobility of the hip joints.

Do not do the exercise if you have sciatica or problems in the lower back or discs.

Conclude with the "corpsepose stretch" (page 70) or "shoulder bridge" (page 71).

Important!

➤ Assume the "seated sun pose" (page 60). Bend the right leg, keeping the foot flat on the mat. Hold the calf with both hands **(1)**.

Exhale, pulling the leg up as high as possible. Let the forehead touch the knee or calf **(2)**. Remain in this position for 10 seconds; the breath is relaxed and even.

Inhale, placing the foot back on the mat. Exhale, low-

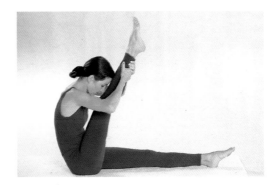

ering the outstretched leg, and letting it rest on the mat.

Repeat the exercise with the left leg.

● Do the exercise, alternating legs, two or three times with both legs.

**Leg stretch
(1), (2)**

Knee-Head Pose

Janu-sirsasana: *Janu* means knee,*sirsa* head.

Effects of the exercise: It stretches the muscles of the back, increases the flexibility of the spine and the hip joints, is helpful when you are tired or nervous, stimulates digestion, and improves breathing.

Exercise with care if you have back or joint pain.

Important! Do not do the exercise if you suffer from acute sciatica, severe problems with the spine, or pain in the groin region.

Conclude with the "corpse-pose stretch" (page 70) or "shoulder bridge" (page 71).

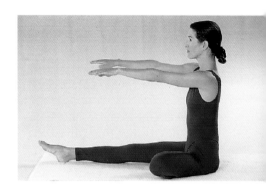

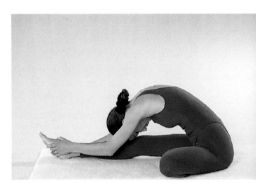

Knee-head pose (1), (2)

▶ Assume the "seated sun pose" (page 60). Spread the legs apart about 23 to 31 in. (60 to 80 cm), and place the left heel in front of the perineum.

Inhale, while lifting both outstretched arms to shoulders' height, with the palms facing down (**1**).

Exhale, bending the upper torso down at the hips over the outstretched right leg. Place the forehead on the knee or the calf. Depending on how flexible you are, reach for and hold on to the toes, foot, or calf with both hands (**2**). Remain in this position for a few breaths; the breath is relaxed and even.

Inhale, returning to the upright seated position. Repeat the exercise with the left leg.

● Do the exercise, alternating sides, two or three times with each leg.

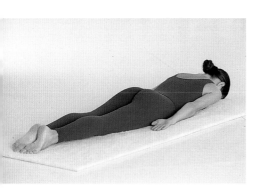

Stomach pose

Stomach Pose

This is the starting position for all asanas that develop from lying on the floor on the stomach.

Effects of the exercise: The stomach pose dissolves overall tension, relieves back pain, and improves breathing.

➤ Lie down on your stomach, with your forehead resting on the mat. The arms are relaxed and alongside the body, the palms facing up. The legs and feet are straight, and the tops of the feet face the mat **(photo).**

Imagine lengthening the entire body by stretching from the top of the head, along the spine, to the toes and the tips of the fingers.

Dolphin

Makarasana: *Makara* means dolphin.

This is the relaxing position following the bending-back exercises: the "half-cobra" (page 54), "cat" (page 55), and "cobra" (page 68).

Effects of the exercise: It deepens breathing, stretches the muscles of the shoulders, arms, and legs, increases the flexibility of the ankles, and is helpful if you have problems with the upper spine.

➤ Assume the "stomach pose" (see left column).

Spread the legs apart about 15 to 19 in. (40 to 50 cm). Allow the inside edge of the feet to rest on the mat, pulling the toes up in the direction of the calves **(1).**

Dolphin (1)

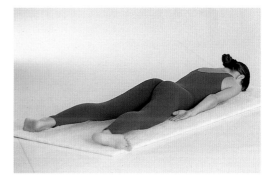

Asanas—Exercises

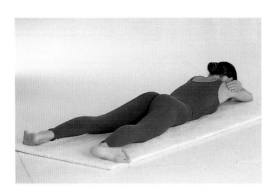

Dolphin (2)   Raise the head, placing the right hand on the left shoulder and the left hand on the right shoulder; then rest the head on the forearms. (**2**).

Lengthen the body, from the elbows up and over the top of the head and from the waist down to the heels. Remain in this position for 60 to 90 seconds.

Return to the starting position.

● Do the exercise once.

Cobra

Bhujangasana: *Bhujanga* means serpent or cobra.

Effects of the exercise: The cobra strengthens the muscles of the upper body, improves flexibility and the alignment of the spine, improves kidney function, and reduces fat deposits in the waist, hips, and thighs.

Do not do the exercise if you have lower-back pain, sciatica, inflammation in the abdominal or reproductive organs, angina pectoris, or a nervous heart condition, or have recently had fractures or surgery.   **Important!**

Conclude with the "corpse-pose stretch" (page 70).

➤ Assume the "stomach pose" (page 67).

Place the hands on the floor at chest height, and stretch the whole body from the top of the head to the toes. Remain in this stretch to the end of the exercise (photo (**1**), page 69). The breath is relaxed and even throughout.

Now raise your head, and—vertebra by vertebra—pull the upper body off the floor, using the muscles of the back. The navel remains in

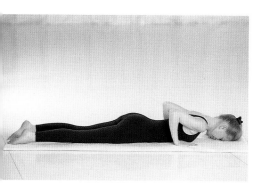

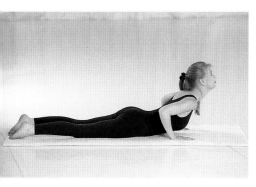

Cobra (1), (2) contact with the floor, and the hands support the body only lightly. Bend back the head and back, stretching the chest upward (**2**). Remember to keep the breath relaxed and even. Remain in this position for three to four breaths. Then slowly return to the starting position.

● Do the exercise two or three times.

Corpse Pose

Effects of the exercise: The corpse pose dissolves tension throughout the body and helps bring about a more complete involvement of the diaphragm and the chest region during breathing.

➤ Lie on your back, with the hands resting alongside the body. Stretch the neck, pulling the chin slightly toward the chest. Gently stretch the legs, which may be 4 to 8 in. (10 to 20 cm) apart. (See **photo** below.)

Imagine the whole body elongating, starting from the top of the head and going down to the tips of the fingers and through the pelvis to the heels and then all the way down to the toes.

■ Conclude all exercise programs in the corpse pose.

Corpse pose

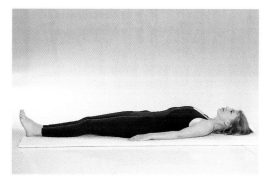

Asanas—Exercises

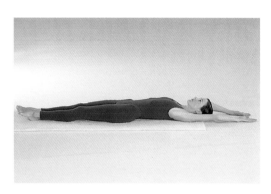

head; then rest the arms on the floor **(photo)**.

Consciously stretch the entire body, from the tips of the fingers down to the toes.

Move the arms back, letting them rest alongside the body. Then rise slowly by rolling over to the right side.

Rebalancing from the Corpse Pose

Apanasana: *Apana* is the prana that affects elimination.

This is a good exercise to do after concluding all exercises entailing bending the body backward, such as the "half-cobra" (page 54), "cat" (page 55), and "cobra" (page 68).

Effects of the exercise: It stimulates digestion and kidney function, and relaxes the back.

Don't forget

▶ Assume the "corpse pose" (page 69).

Bend the legs, and pull them toward the upper body. Hold the calves with both hands.

At each exhalation, pull the legs close to the body (photo **(1)**, page 71).

Alternative corpse-pose stretch

Corpse-Pose Stretch

Assume this alternative relaxation pose after completing all strenuous asanas, such as the "full bend" (page 51), "half spinal twist" (page 64), "leg stretch" (page 65), "knee-head pose" (page 66), and "plow" (page 74).

Effects of the exercise: It relaxes and refreshes the entire body and is helpful if you have painful muscle tension or are exhausted.

▶ Assume the "corpse pose" (page 69).

Imagine being supported by the ground. Let go of all tension in the muscles. Allow the breath to flow freely. Remain in this position for about 30 to 60 seconds.

Inhale, while lifting your outstretched arms over your

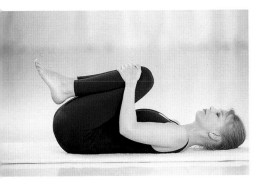

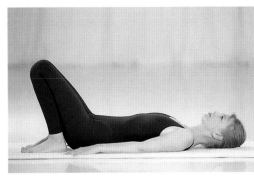

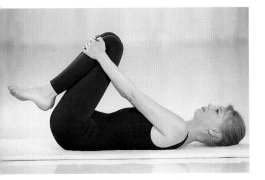

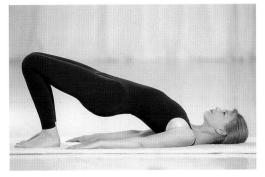

Rebalancing from the corpse pose (1), (2)

Allow the legs to move out with each inhalation as far as the arms will allow (2). The hands always remain in the same place on the calves.

You can improve the quality of the exercise by increasingly fine-tuning the leg and arm movements.

● Do the exercise about 10 times.

Shoulder Bridge

Dvipada pitham: *Dvi* means two, *pada* means river, and *pitham* means desk.

The shoulder bridge is a good rebalancing exercise to do after concluding all the exercises that require bending forward, such as the "full bend" (page 51), "leg stretch" (page 65), "knee-head pose" (page 66), "plow" (page 74), and "roll" (page 77).

Shoulder bridge (1), (2)

Asanas—Exercises

Effects of the exercise: The shoulder bridge deepens breathing, strengthens the legs and back, and stretches the muscles in the front of the body.

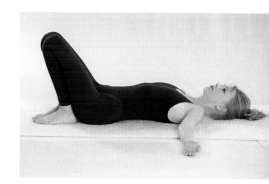

➤ Assume the "corpse pose" (page 69).

Place the feet as close to the buttocks as possible, knees touching (photo (**1**), page 71). Push with the soles of the feet, lifting the buttocks off the floor (photo (**2**), page 71). Remain in this position for one to two minutes; the breath is relaxed and even.

● Do the exercise once.

This asana can be expanded with the following breathing exercise:

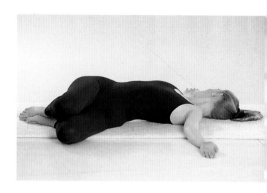

Breathing exercise

➤ Move the stretched-out arms behind your head while inhaling and back again while exhaling.

● Do this exercise five or six times.

Crocodile

Nakrasana: *Nakra* means crocodile.

Effects of the exercise: It increases the flexibility of the spine and back, dissolves tension in the shoulders, back, and hips, supports the functions of the digestive organs, deepens breathing, stimulates the metabolism, and strengthens the nerves.

Crocodile (1), (2)

Important! Do not do this exercise if you are having problems with the vertebrae of the spine.

➤ Assume the "corpse pose" (page 69). The outstretched arms are placed on the floor at shoulders' height, the palms facing up.

Bend the legs, and place them as close to the buttocks as possible, knees touching (photo **(1)**, page 72). Let the legs fall gently to the mat on the left side, while turning your head to the right; the breath is relaxed and even (photo **(2)**, page 72). With the next inhalation, lift the legs off the floor, and—while exhaling—move them to the right side in one fluid motion, as you turn your head to the left.

● Do the exercise five or six times.

Leg Lift

Urdhva prasrita padasana: *Urdhva* means upward, *prasrita* means outstretched, and *pada* means leg.

Effects of the exercise: The leg lift strengthens the muscles of the lower back and legs, compensates for a hollow back, and prevents sciatica.

Do not do the exercise if you have acute sciatica or if there is any damage to the spine or the discs in the lumbar region.

➤ Assume the "corpse pose" (page 69), with the arms outstretched alongside the body, palms down.

In a semi-circle, move the outstretched arms vertically, placing them on the mat above your head. Exhale and by tensing the muscles of the abdomen and the legs, pull the bent legs above the upper body **(1)**.

Stretch the legs to the ceiling, while—in a fluid motion—moving the outstretched arms in a semi-circle back to alongside the body (photo **(2)**, page 74). Remain in this position for 10 seconds; the breath is relaxed and even.

Leg lift (1)

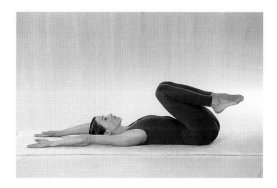

Asanas—Exercises

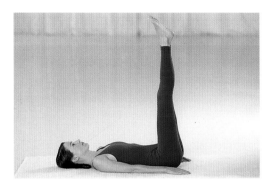

Leg lift (2)

Then move the legs back to the mat with one breath.

● Do the exercise three times.

Plow

Halasana: *Hala* means plow.
Effects of the exercise: The plow has many benefits. It stretches the spine and the muscles of the upper body, relieves tension and tension headaches, increases circulation in the brain, improves the complexion, strengthens the abductor muscles of the legs, reduces fat deposits in the buttocks and thighs, stimulates the functions of the liver, stomach, pancreas, intestine, and kidneys, and relieves fatigue.

Do not do the exercise if you have a tightening of the spine or acute sciatica, if there is a danger of elevated ocular pressure or a detached retina, or after recent surgery or fractures.

Conclude with the "corpse-pose stretch" (page 70) or "shoulder bridge" (page 71).

➤ Assume the "corpse pose," with the arms at the sides, the palms down (page 69).

Lightly push the fingers down, engage the muscles of the abdomen and the legs, and move the legs at a right angle above the upper body.

Plow (1)

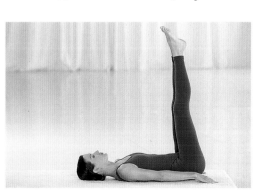

Plow (2)

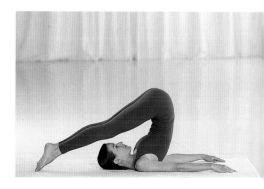

The legs are then stretched out, with the toes pointing to the ceiling (photo (1), page 74).

In a continuous movement, lower the legs gently over your head, as the spine lifts off the mat one vertebra at a time. The knees are slightly bent as they sink toward the face, allowing the back to be well rounded. Let the toes touch the floor behind your head. Now gently push the feet as far away from your head as possible (photo (2), page 74). Remain in this position for about 30 to 60 seconds; the breath is relaxed and even.

● Do this exercise two or three times.

Half Shoulder Stand (and Shoulder Stand)

Viparita-karani-sarvangasana: *Viparita* means reverse, *karana* movement, and *sarvanga* the whole body.

Effects of the exercise: This exercise influences the whole body in a very positive way, as the following quote makes clear:

"Sarvangasana is the mother of all asanas. Like a mother creating harmony and joy in the family, this asana seeks to create joy and harmony for the human body. It is the universal healing remedy for most ordinary ailments."

—B. K. S. Iyengar, *Light and Yoga*

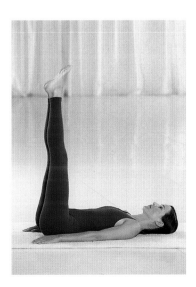

Half shoulder stand (1)

Asanas—Exercises

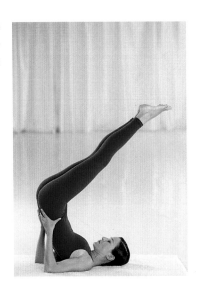

Do not do the exercise if you have problems in the spinal column, increased ocular pressure or detachment of the retina, asthma, heart problems, high blood pressure, impaired balance, or recent fractures, if you are considerably overweight, or during menstruation or advanced pregnancy (after five months).

▶ Assume the "corpse pose" (page 69), with the arms at the sides, the palms down.

Support yourself lightly with the hands and forearms, and engage the stomach and leg muscles as you pull the bent legs toward and over the upper body. Exhale and raise the legs up vertically (photo (1), page 75). Let the legs' sink slowly into a horizontal position, allowing the back to come off the mat one vertebra at a time.

Place both hands at the waist, the thumbs pointing down and the upper arms parallel to each other.

Lift the legs halfway between vertical and horizontal—this is the half shoulder stand (2). Remain in this position as long as it is comfortable. The breath is relaxed and even.

Pull the buttocks up, letting the chin touch the chest. When the back, buttocks, and legs are in a straight line, you are in the shoulder stand position. The hands are now supporting the upper back (photo **(3)**, page 76).

Remain in this position for just a few seconds, and increase the amount over time. Make sure that the breath is relaxed and even.

Return to the "corpse pose" by reversing the order of the steps.

Make it easy for yourself

● Suggestion: Place a folded blanket under the shoulders in such a way that the fold of the blanket and the upper edge of the shoulders are lined up. This relieves pressure from the neck and head, making the shoulders carry the weight of the body, as intended.

Roll

Effects of the exercise: It massages and relaxes the neck and back, increases the flexibility of the spinal column, stimulates circulation, increases vitality, and combats exhaustion.

Do not do the exercise if you have severe back problems or if your spinal column is restricted.

Conclude with the "shoulder bridge" (page 71).

Roll (1), (2)

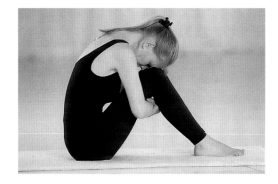

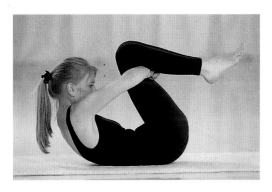

Asanas—Exercises

▶ Sit on a soft mat with the legs bent and close together. Fold the forearms around the thighs behind the knees, letting your head rest on the knees (photo (**1**), page 77).

Shift your weight back, and gently roll on your back; then use your momentum to move back into the sitting position (photo (**2**), page 77). Keep the distance between the head and the knees as close as possible.

● Roll back and forth several times carefully and gently.

Relaxing on the Wall

Effects of the exercise: It supports the flow of the blood back to the heart and is helpful if you have varicose veins or hemorrhoids.

Even helpful for hemorrhoids

▶ With bent legs, sit as close to a wall as possible (photo (**1**)).

Lie down on the back. Raise the legs up, the heels touching the wall (photo (**2**)). Remain in this position for several minutes, while you stretch up from the top of the head, down at the fingertips, and up at the toes.

You can expand on the exercise by imagining-as you inhale—the color red flowing from the pelvis through the legs and up to the toes and—as you exhale—the color blue flowing back the same way.

Stretch out on the mat for one to two minutes, allowing the blood to flow back to the legs; then roll to one side and get up.

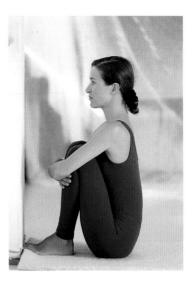

Relaxing on the wall (1)

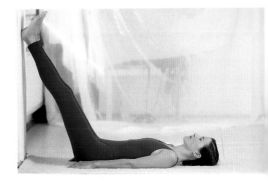

Relaxing on the wall (2)

Yoga Deep Relaxation

Finding peace

Proper relaxation is an active, wide-awake, and focused process that involves the body, mind, and emotions. This cooperative practice is important, because it is only when burdensome feelings or thoughts are allowed to come to rest that it is possible to dissolve deep-seated physical and emotional tensions and reach true relaxation.

■ Always finish your daily yoga program with a relaxation exercise. It's the best way to lessen emotional worries without denying them. Being fully present means having more peace, increased freedom, and greater composure.

➤ Assume the "corpse pose" (page 69). Spread the legs 7 to 11 in. (20 to 30 cm) apart. If you have pain in the back, bend the legs; for pain in the neck, lie on a small pillow.

Feel your entire body stretching, from the head upward, from the pelvis down to the heels and toes, and also down at the fingertips. This is the first step in relieving muscle tension.

Close your eyes; the breath is relaxed and even. Observe your breath without trying to influence it. With every exhalation, dissolve internal and external tension. Start at the head. With special tenderness, relax the eyelids, the mouth, and the muscles of the jaw. Let the teeth touch without pressure; the mouth is closed, and the tongue relaxed and resting at the bottom of the lower jaw.

Release tension

Concentrate on the neck. With each exhalation, release any tension. Move to the shoulders, arms, and hands-in these places, too, let go of any tension as you exhale.

Relax the chest, waist, pelvis, legs, and feet in the same way.

For a few moments, observe the free-flowing breath and the calmness in the body. This is yoga deep relaxation, and will divert your mind from troublesome thoughts and free your soul.

Here is how to conclude the relaxation exercise:

Deepen exhalation

➤ Increase the exhalation for a few breaths. With every inhalation, raise the arms over your head and stretch from the fingertips down to the toes.

Return the arms to the sides; turn to the right—to

avoid restricting the heart—and raise yourself off the mat.

■ Once you have mastered yoga deep relaxation, you can combine it with "awakening energies" on page 32.

Putting a Program Together

In order to avoid repetition, the exercises in this book are not organized according to a program but instead are arranged according to the respective starting positions. On the following pages (81–83) are eight exercise program in increasing degrees of difficulty.

Each program takes about 20 to 30 minutes and exercises the entire body. Alternative and relaxation positions are integrated in the programs, so that you can avoid overtaxing individual muscle groups. Start with Program I. Do each program every day for as long as it takes to master it. Depending on your flexibility and condition, this may take anywhere from one to four weeks. Only then should you move on to the next program.

If you are already familiar with the exercises and have experience with yoga, you may put together your own program from the exercises provided in the book. But be sure that the program is well balanced and, if necessary, includes alternative poses.

When a relaxation exercise is called for, you will find the relevant information on the page where the exercise begins. Always conclude your program with a relaxation exercise.

Take note of rebalancing exercises

Program/Name and Exercises	Page	How Often/ How Long
Program I		
Relaxing at the wall	78	a few minutes
Upright position	41	about 15 seconds
Tree I	43	2 or 3 times each side
Leaning half-moon	45	2 or 3 times each side, alternating sides
Side triangle	47	2 or 3 times each side, alternating sides
Corpse-pose stretch	70	1 to 2 minutes
Increasing flexibility	61	4 to 6 times each side
Tailor's seat	61	about 1 minute
Yoga deep relaxation	79	5 to 10 minutes
Program II		
Relaxing on the wall	78	a few minutes
Roll	77	about 1 minute
Leg stretch	65	2 or 3 times each side
Cat	55	3 or 4 times each side
Blade	59	3 to 5 times
Upright position	41	about 15 seconds
Pendulum	42	2 or 3 times
Full bend	51	twice
Shoulder bridge	71	about 1 minute
Yoga deep relaxation	79	5 to 10 minutes
Program III		
Relaxation on the wall	78	about 15 seconds
Stretched hand-toe pose	50	2 to 3 times each side
Full bend	51	3 times
Corpse-pose stretch	70	about 1 minute
Leg lift	73	3 times
Half shoulder stand	75	15 to 30 seconds
Shoulder bridge	71	about 1 minute
Yoga deep relaxation	79	5 to 10 minutes

Asanas—Exercises

Program/Name and Exercises	Page	How Often/ How Long
Program IV		
Relaxing on the wall	78	a few minutes
Squat I	44	3 to 8 times
Flower	58	3 times
Half spinal twist	64	2 or 3 times each side
Upright position	41	about 15 seconds
Tree I	43	2 or 3 times each side
Hero	49	15 to 20 seconds each side
Twisting triangle	48	4 times each side
Yoga deep relaxation	79	5 to 10 minutes
Program V		
Relaxing on the wall	78	a few minutes
Leg stretch	65	2 times
Knee-head pose	66	2 times each side
Heel-seat position	56	1 time
Baby pose	57	20 to 30 seconds
Upright position	41	about 15 seconds
Tree II	46	2 or 3 times each side
Full bend	51	2 times
Yoga deep relaxation	79	5 to 10 minutes
Program VI		
Relaxing on the wall	78	a few minutes
Half-Cobra	54	2 or 3 times
Corpse-pose stretch	70	about 30 seconds
Heel-seat position	56	once
Mountain variation	63	20 to 30 seconds
Upright position	41	about 15 seconds
Twisting triangle	48	4 times each side
Squat II	49	2 or 3 times
Dolphin	67	2 or 3 times
Yoga deep relaxation	79	5 to 10 minutes

Program/Name and Exercises	Page	How Often/ How Long
Program VII		
Relaxing on the wall	78	a few minutes
Increasing flexibility	61	4 to 6 times each side
Tailor's seat	61	once
Cat	55	2 or 3 times each side
Half-cobra	54	2 or 3 times
Cobra	68	2 or 3 times
Corps-pose stretch	70	6 to 10 times
Crocodile	72	5 or 6 times each side
Yoga deep relaxation	79	5 to 10 minutes
Program VIII		
Relaxing on the wall	78	a few minutes
Half spinal twist	64	2 or 3 times each side
Lion	57	2 times
Baby pose	57	20 to 30 seconds
Plow	74	2 times
Half shoulder stand	75	15 to 30 seconds
Shoulder stand	75	once
Shoulder bridge	71	once
Yoga deep relaxation	79	5 to 10 minutes

Relaxing "In Between"

Dissolving tension

All of us would like to be able to relax effectively during stressful or tiring situations.

Each of the following exercises will help you dissolve emotional and physical tension during the course of a day. You might also consider integrating some of these exercises into your daily yoga program. It's important to carry out these exercises with the same care and attention that you give to the asanas. Furthermore, make sure that the breath, movement, and concentration coalesce, thereby bringing into balance the body, mind, and emotions.

Relaxing the Eyes

The following three exercises are helpful in quickly relaxing tired eyes. They are especially useful for those of us who work long hours on the computer or take long trips by car.

Near and Far Distance

Effects of the exercise: It relaxes the eyes and the muscles surrounding the eyes.

➤ Hold one hand about 6 in., or 15 cm, in front of your eyes. Observe every detail of the palm for about 15 seconds **(photo)**.

Move the hand to the side, and concentrate looking into the far distance.

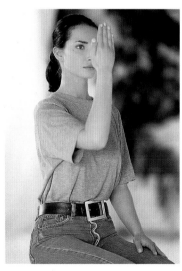

Near and far distance

● Do this exercise five or six times. Then rub your hands together to warm the palms, and place them for 15 seconds on top of the closed eyelids.

Eye Circles

Effects of the exercise: Eye circles relax the muscles around the eyes and have a calming effect on the entire nervous system.

➤ Imagine that a large clock with huge numbers is in front of your eyes very close—the face of the clock is larger than your face.

Take your time

Without raising your head, look at 12 o'clock. Now let your eyes glide effortlessly and without stopping from number to number until you reach 12 once more.

The exercise should take about 30 seconds.

Then do the same in a counterclockwise direction.

● Do the exercise two or three times.

● Further relax the eyes and the muscles surrounding them by rubbing your hands together to warm the palms and placing them over the closed eyelids.

Pressure on the Eyes

Effects of the exercise: This exercise balances the functions of the internal organs.

➤ Close your eyes. Imagine that you are looking with closed eyes straight ahead.

With the tip of the index finger, explore one eye under the closed lid; then press the tip of the finger gently on the eye for about 15 seconds **(photo).**

● Do the exercise once on both eyes.

● Relax the eyes and the muscles surrounding them by rubbing your hands together

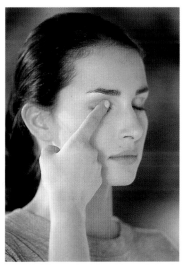

Pressure on the eyes

to warm the palms and placing them on top of the closed eyelids.

Relaxing the Ears

Tension in the jaw muscles can lead to tension in and around the ears. Massaging the ears will help.

Ear Massage

Effects of the exercise: The ear massage dissolves tension in the ears.

➤ Hold the ears between the thumbs and the bent index fingers. Apply a good amount of pressure, as you

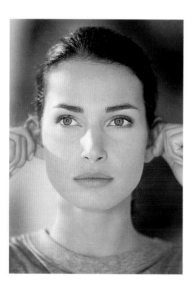

Ear massage

massage both ears at the same time for 60 to 90 seconds **(photo)**.

● Do the exercise once.

Relaxing the Tongue

With the following three exercises, you can influence the stomach and the pancreas by way of the esophagus. Tension in the tongue prevents the diaphragm from moving down far enough into the abdomen during inhalation. Often the tongue presses against the palate or the teeth when tense. A relaxed tongue will lie loosely in the "bowl" of the lower jaw.

Improves breathing

Exploring the Oral Cavity

Effects of the exercise: It relaxes the muscles of the head and fosters natural, complete breathing.

➤ Explore the inside of the closed mouth with the tip of the tongue for about 30 to 60 seconds. Let the tip of the tongue stay for 15 seconds at the places on the palate where it is closest to the eyes. Experience the relaxing, comforting effect on the eyes.

Be careful: Dentures may come loose during this exercise.

Sucking on a Lemon

Quick result

Effects of the exercise: This exercise is helpful if your mouth feels dry. In addition to increasing the flow of saliva, it supports digestion.

➤ Act as if a slice of lemon is in your mouth and you are sucking on it. Do so for 30 seconds.

● Do this exercise two times.

Exploring Your Teeth

Effects of the exercise: This exercise relaxes the muscles in the mouth cavity and the tongue, stimulates the flow of saliva and aids digestion, and improves the flexibility of the diaphragm.

➤ With the tip of the tongue, cautiously explore the outside of the teeth in the upper jaw and then the teeth in the lower jaw. Be careful: Dentures may come loose or shift.

● Do the exercise a few times, alternating going from right to left and from left to right.

● This exercise increases the flow of saliva, which you can swallow at the end of the exercise to stimulate digestion.

Relaxing the Neck and Shoulders

The neck area is where misfortune often hits us the hardest, and indeed the muscles in the neck and the shoulders are often tensed up and painful. Tension in the neck and the shoulders is frequently the cause of headaches, poor blood circulation in the

Relaxing the neck

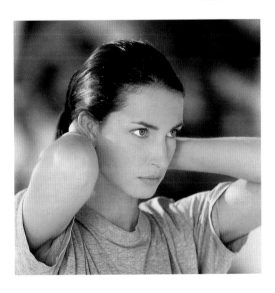

arms and hands, ringing in the ears, dizziness, and visual difficulties.

Relaxing the Neck

Effects of the exercise: This exercise strengthens weak neck muscles.

➤ Lace your fingers, and place them in the back of the neck. Push as hard against the fingers with the neck muscles as you can. Push the fingers into the neck at the same time. (See **photo** on page 85.) Keep the tension for 15 seconds. Release the pressure evenly.

● Do the exercise three times.

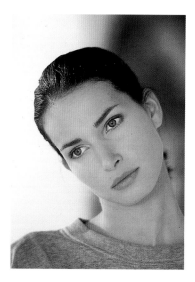

Head bending

Head Bending

Effects of the exercise: Head bending stretches tense neck muscles.

➤ Bend your head to the right side, pushing down the left shoulder; observe how the muscles on the left side of the neck are being stretched. Remain in this position for about 20 seconds **(photo)**.
 Then bend the head to the left side, pushing down the right shoulder. Again, remain in this position for about 20 seconds.
 Next, bend your head back and then forward, holding each position for about 20 seconds.

● Do the side bending and the back and forward bending alternately two times.

Head Circles

Effects of the exercise: Head circles relax the muscles of the head, neck, and shoulders.

➤ Allow your head to sink forward, and with an inhalation start to rotate your head slowly back and over the left shoulder and with the exhalation slowly forward (see **photo** on page 89). With the

Exercise with care

Head circles

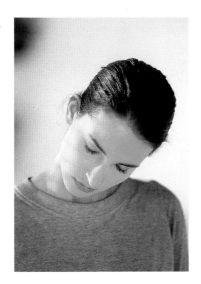

arms relaxed next to the body, the palms facing the thighs. In a flowing motion, turn the palms back and then to the outside until the backs of the hands face the thighs. Remain in this position for about 30 seconds.

In a flowing motion, rotate the palms back and beyond the original position so that they now face the outside. Again, remain in this position for about 30 seconds.

● Do this exercise two or three times with both hands.

Shoulder Rolls

Effects of the exercise: Shoulder rolls relax tension in the neck, shoulder region, and upper back.

next inhalation, do the same, but this time back and over the right shoulder and with the exhalation slowly forward again. The circle is not completed, because this would overtax the neck vertebrae.

● Start by doing three open circles, increasing the number depending on how comfortable you are. Observe how the head movement and the breath begin to merge.

Shoulder Relaxation

Effects of the exercise: This exercise dissolves tension in the neck, shoulders, and arms.

➤ Stand upright, with the

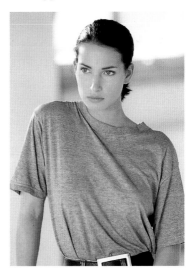

Shoulder rolls

Allow the arms to be relaxed at your sides. Roll the right shoulder several times forward and then back (**photo**).

Concentrate on how the tips of the fingers move with each circle. Then roll the left shoulder. Conclude with rotating both shoulders together in both directions.

● Do the exercise for each shoulder five times.

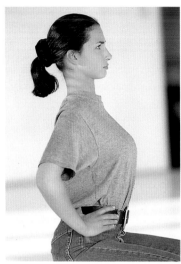

Pelvis rock (1)

Relaxing the Pelvic Region

Easy remedy

Tension in the pelvic girdle can cause backaches, sciatica, and pain in the hips. You can find relief with the following exercises.

Pelvis Rock

Effects of the exercise: This exercise dissolves tension in the pelvis and lower back, and prevents pain due to sciatica.

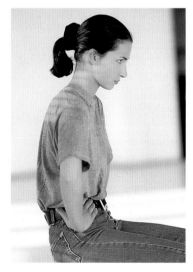

Pelvis rock (2)

➤ Sit upright on a chair or a cushion, and rock the upper part of the pelvis forward (**1**) and then back (**2**). The upper body remains straight. Expand the movement by imagining pushing the navel out horizontally and a lumbar vertebra back horizontally. Do the exercise in this exaggerated manner.

● Move the pelvis for about 60 seconds in rhythm with your breath, inhaling forward and exhaling backward.

Pelvis Rotation

Effects of the exercise: The pelvis rotation relaxes muscles in the lower back, pelvis, and thighs, brings relief to the lumbar spine, and increases flexibility.

➤ It is an expansion of the previous exercise. Imagine that you are sitting on the face of a clock with the number 12 at your coccyx bone. Now shift your weight in such a way that a rotating movement touches every number on the face of the clock. The upper body remains upright. Start at the number 12.

● Rotate several times in each direction.

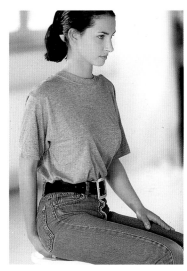

Turning the pelvis upright

Turning the Pelvis Upright

Effects of the exercise: This exercise moves the pelvis to an upright position.

➤ Sit upright on a chair. Place the left hand under the left buttock with the fingers pointing forward. Balance your weight equally over the buttocks, and pull the hand back and out from under you (photo).

● Do the exercise once on each side.

Relaxation Exercises at a Glance			
Complaints	Exercise	Page	How Long/ How Often
Burning eyes	Near & far distance	84	5 or 6 times
	Ear massage	86	about 60 seconds
Tired eyes & facial tension	Eye circles	85	2 times in both directions
Emotional tension	Pressure on the eyes	85	2 times in both directions
	Ear massage	86	about 60 seconds
Head tension	Ear massage	86	about 60 seconds
	Head bending	88	about 20 seconds in each direction
	Head circles	88	3 times in each direction
	Exploring your teeth	87	20 to 30 seconds
	Exploring the oral cavity	86	about 60 seconds
Tongue tightness	Exploring your teeth	87	20 to 30 your seconds
	Exploring the oral cavity	86	about 60 seconds
Dry mouth	Sucking on a lemon	87	about 60 seconds
Tense neck	Ear massage	86	about 60 seconds
	Head bending	88	about 20 seconds in each direction
	Head circles	88	3 times in each direction
	Relaxing the neck	88	3 times for 15 seconds each
Tense neck	Head circles	88	3 times in each direction

Relaxation Exercises at a Glance

Complaints	Exercise	Page	How Long/ How Often
Tense shoulders	Shoulder rolls	89	5 times in each direction
	Head circles	88	3 times in each direction
	Head bending	88	about 20 seconds in each direction
Tense arms	Shoulder relaxation	89	2 to 3 times in each direction
	Shoulder rolls	89	5 times in each direction
Tense pelvis	Ear massage	86	about 60 seconds
	Pelvis rock	90	6 to 8 times, increasing over time
	Turning the pelvis upright	91	once on each side
Tense diaphragm	Exploring the oral cavity	86	about 30 seconds
	Exploring your teeth	87	20 to 30 seconds
	Ear massage	86	about 60 seconds
	Pelvis rock	90	6 to 8 times, increasing over time
	Pelvis rotation	90	2 times in each direction

About This Book

Yoga—a centuries-old system of exercises from India—can be helpful in releasing physical and emotional tension, finding peace and serenity, and developing self-confidence. Unlike any other method, yoga reduces everyday stress and diminishes—and, when practiced consistently, may even prevent—the negative consequences of today's hectic lifestyles.

One of the forms most widely practiced is hatha yoga, which combines breathing, physical movement, and metal concentration. Hatha yoga improves stamina, alertness, health, and overall well-being.

The author, an experienced yoga teacher, wrote this book specifically for the beginner. He explains breathing exercises (pranayamas) for natural, complete breathing, physical exercises (asanas) to harmonize the whole body, and tension-releasing exercises. The hatha yoga exercises presented in this book can be performed by everyone, regardless of age.

Every phase of the exercises is clearly explained and illustrated. The eight successive programs build on each other, making it easy for the beginner to learn this method, step by step.

Yoga will help you to live every day happier and more fully.

About the Author

Harry Waesse, born in 1934, has been a health practitioner and a yoga teacher since 1975. He has taught at many community colleges and at the Yoga-Center in Munich, and continues to participate in yoga seminars offered by German as well as foreign yoga teachers. In his holistic practice, he combines hatha yoga with breathing therapy.

Index